CORE TEACHING PRACTICES for HEALTH EDUCATION

Phillip Ward, PhD

The Ohio State University

Shonna Snyder, PhD

Gardner-Webb University

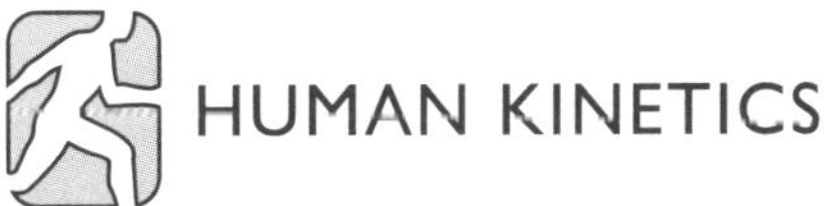

HUMAN KINETICS

Library of Congress Cataloging-in-Publication Data

Names: Ward, Phillip, 1957- author. | Snyder, Shonna L., 1973- author.
Title: Core teaching practices for health education / Phillip Ward, PhD,
  The Ohio State University, Shonna L. Snyder, PhD, Gardner-Webb
  University.
Description: Champaign, IL : Human Kinetics, Inc. [2022] | Includes
  bibliographical references.
Identifiers: LCCN 2021016293 (print) | LCCN 2021016294 (ebook) | ISBN
  9781492597810 (paperback) | ISBN 9781492597827 (epub) | ISBN
  9781492597834 (pdf)
Subjects: LCSH: Health education--Study and teaching--United States.
Classification: LCC RA440.3.U5 W28 2022 (print) | LCC RA440.3.U5 (ebook)
  | DDC 613.071--dc23
LC record available at https://lccn.loc.gov/2021016293
LC ebook record available at https://lccn.loc.gov/2021016294
ISBN: 978-1-4925-9781-0 (print)

The web addresses cited in this text were current as of April 2022, unless otherwise noted.

Acquisitions Editor: Bethany J. Bentley; **Developmental Editor:** Anne Hall; **Managing Editor:** Melissa J. Zavala; **Copyeditor:** Marissa Wold Uhrina; **Proofreader:** Rodelinde Albrecht; **Permissions Manager:** Dalene Reeder; **Graphic Designer:** Julie L. Denzer; **Cover Designer:** Julie L. Denzer; **Art Director:** Keri Evans; **Cover Design Specialist:** Susan Rothermel Allen; **Photograph (cover):** © fizkes/iStockphoto/Getty Images; © SDI Productions/E+/Getty Images; **Photo Production Manager:** Jason Allen; **Photo Asset Manager:** Laura Fitch; **Senior Art Manager:** Kelly Hendren; **Illustrations:** © Human Kinetics; **Printer:** Versa Press

Printed in the United States of America   10 9 8 7 6 5 4 3 2 1

The paper in this book is certified under a sustainable forestry program.

Human Kinetics
1607 N. Market Street
Champaign, IL 61820
USA

United States and International	*Canada*
Website: **US.HumanKinetics.com**	Website: **Canada.HumanKinetics.com**
Email: info@hkusa.com	Email: info@hkcanada.com
Phone: 1-800-747-4457	

E8058

Tell us what you think!
Human Kinetics would love to hear what we
can do to improve the customer experience.
Use this QR code to take our brief survey.

Contents

PART III   **Growing as a Teacher**

Preface

Teachers make a difference. Moreover, teachers are the best and most cost-effective means of improving the education of children in PreK-12 schools. But the task of teaching is challenging. Among the largest challenges for health educators is taking curriculum content in health education, determining what is meaningful for students, and aligning it to health standards, then teaching that content in ways that connect to students in ways that promote understanding, skill development, and decision-making.

Conceptions of effective teaching and of quality health teaching have changed markedly over the past decade. Historically, effective teachers have been viewed as decision makers who apply professional and subject-specific knowledge. Recent conceptions of effective teaching have emphasized the use of a teacher's professional judgment in two ways. First, emphasis on adapting instruction has increased, not just in the planning stages of teaching but during the act of teaching, by modifying instruction and focusing on the representation of the content of the lesson in response to student understandings or misunderstandings. Second, the scope of health education, like many subject areas in the 21st century, is so broad that teachers require skills that allow them to judge how to organize the content using concepts like big ideas (chapter 2), enduring understandings (chapter 3), and essential questions (chapter 4) to drive, connect, and progress students' health understandings skills and decision-making. *Core Teaching Practices for Health Education* presents 21st-century teaching skills as core practices specific to health education.

Our purpose in writing this book is to provide preservice teachers, in-service teachers, and teacher educators with the core practices of teaching health education. Our goals are to

1. provide explanation and rationale for core practices of teaching health education,
2. situate these core practices of teaching health education within the practice-based teacher education movement,
3. provide clear guidance on how to use these core practices in health classrooms, and
4. support teacher efforts in using core teaching practices to address the big ideas in health education.

While core practices are effective and can be taught to teachers, one challenge is that because core practices require specific understandings and guidance, they are seldom acquired by experience alone. Throughout a teacher's career they might only discover a handful of core practices. However, a critical characteristic of core practices is that they allow teachers to learn more about their students and about their own teaching as they make decisions about when and how to use each practice. In short, teachers are able grow their teaching skills with practice. A second critical characteristic of core practices is that because they are not tied to any one health content area, standard, or grade level, they are highly transferable across curricula because they require teacher decision-making.

In the past decade, other subject areas such as music, math, science, and history have shown a focus on core teaching practices aligned to each subject matter (Ball, Sleep, Boerst, and Bass 2009; Fogo 2014; Grossman et al. 2009; Kloser 2014; Schneider Kavanagh , Shahan, and Morrison 2017; Windschitl et al. 2018). To date, no core practices have been proposed for health education. In fact, at the time of this writing we could find no reference to the concept or use of core practices in the professional or research literature in health education. This not only places health education out of sync with the larger educational movements in support of teachers, but it also presents a potential barrier to student learning and, we would also argue, the quality of the teaching life that a teacher experiences. In using the term *quality of the teaching life*, we argue that the better the teacher is able to teach, the greater the professional enjoyment and self-worth that teacher will experience. This was recently reported by the American Federation of Teachers 2017 Educator Quality of Work Life survey.

Core Teaching Practices for Health Education provides support for preservice and practicing health education teachers as well as for health teacher educators. In this book, we present core practices for health education teaching. These teaching practices can be used by teachers to improve their students' learning and in turn their own quality of life. Our choices for core practices are based on our collective experiences as health teacher educators and the extensive pedagogical literature in support of core practices in general education (Ball et al. 2009; Council for Exceptional Children 2017; Fogo 2014; Grossman et al. 2009; Kloser 2014; Schneider Kavanagh et al. 2017; Windschitl et al. 2018).

Core Teaching Practices for Health Education begins with an introduction to the idea of core practices and situates them within contemporary education practice and policy. We have organized core practices of teaching health education into three parts. The first focuses on planning for the teaching of health education content. The second part discusses the pedagogy of health education. The third part addresses reflective practices that represent the essential practices from the first two parts. Each core practice has its own chapter.

Each chapter introducing a core practice for health education includes a vignette that illustrates the use of the core practice. We then provide an explanation and rationale for and examples of the core practices. Finally, we provide clear guidance on how to use each core practice in health classrooms. *Core Teaching Practices for Health Education* can be used as a pedagogical guide for teacher educators and as a supporting pedagogical resource in health education methods classes, or the book can be used as a pedagogical resource for practicing teachers and in student teaching for preservice teachers.

Core practices are knowledge and skills to help teachers, particularly beginning teachers, navigate successfully the complex, relational, and contextual nature of teaching. They are also a way for teacher educators to prioritize teaching outcomes in the curriculum. Core practices represent important knowledge and skills so that teachers avoid teaching in a one-size-fits-all manner (i.e., normatively) and instead adapt their instruction to the needs of their students. Adapting instruction to meet student needs is not just a central practice of good teaching, it is an example of equity-centered instruction.

Planning for Teaching

Improving Your Effectiveness Using Core Practices for Teaching Health Education

Teaching health education is complex, relational, and contextual. It is complex in that teachers must make numerous decisions in a lesson because they manage many moving parts in a class period. These moving parts include teacher instruction, the organization and management of the class, responding to student work products, providing feedback, and the like. It is also complex in terms of the knowledge that a teacher must bring to bear in meeting students' needs in a subject area that is substantive in scope and often changing. Among the largest challenges health education teachers face is how to present the content in such a way that it is relevant for students.

Teaching health education is relational because teaching at its simplest level involves interactions between teachers and students and among students. Positive interactions establish and maintain student cooperation in the classroom in order to create a respectful community where learning can occur. Central to the notion of being relational is meeting students where they are in terms of their readiness for learning.

Finally, teaching is contextual because a teacher must take into account the prior work and knowledge of the students. As such, teachers must understand who their students are, personalize students' learning, and view students' readiness in terms of both the class and the individual. Teaching is also contextual because teachers must consider the social and physical environment of the classroom. The space within which teachers must be relational, assess prior knowledge of students, and manage the lesson can affect the success of a particular day. For example, an unkempt space or an imbalance in the classroom's social environment can have a negative impact on a teacher's success.

Teachers make a difference, but effective teachers make even more of a difference. Consider these rankings in table 1.1 from standardized tests in several subjects' data reported by Marzano (2010, p. 214).

TABLE 1.1   **The Relationship Between Teacher Competence and Student Achievement**

Teacher competence on a scale of 1 to 100 percentile	Predicted student learning in relation to teacher competence
50th	50th
70th	58th
90th	68th
98th	77th

The first column shows teachers at the 50th, 70th, 90th, and 98th percentiles of competence. The second column shows the scores of the students on standardized tests as a function of the growing competence of the teacher. Therefore, a teacher at the 50th percentile produces learning gains in students at the 50th percentile. A teacher with the same students (i.e., at the 50th percentile of achievement when with a teacher at the 50th percentile of competence) but who has a higher competence level (e.g., 70th, 90th, and 98th percentiles) produces the gains shown in the righthand column. In short, more effective teachers make more of a difference. This book is a manual for teachers to increase their effectiveness in teaching health education. The material in any one chapter, used as described, will improve teacher effectiveness. Using the material in all of the chapters will improve teaching in profound ways.

Given this description of teaching health education, it is daunting for teachers to navigate successfully the complex, relational, and contextual nature of teaching. In chapter 2 of this book we introduce an important organization concept called *big ideas*. A big idea is a way to package all essential knowledge in ways that allow individuals to make sense of the issues. In thinking about the teaching of health education in preK-12 health education we propose 10 big ideas.

10 Big Ideas of Health Education

The 10 big ideas that follow are a response to critiques that health education is fragmented in its organization and to the pressing problems of health education of preK-12 students. While each state in the United States has established a set of health standards (i.e., 50 sets of standards), most have handed control of the health education curriculum to school districts. There are more than 13,000 school districts, and most teach health uniquely in terms of what they emphasize, what textbook they use (if they use one at all), and the amount of time devoted to health education instruction. The result of this fragmentation is frustration and confusion for health education teachers. The 10 big ideas are meant to set direction for the profession and to create relationships and common understanding in policy and practice.

Idea 1: Support the Whole School, Whole Child, Whole Community Model

Throughout the years of preK-12 education, schools should, through their health education curricula, support the five tenets of the Whole School, Whole Child, Whole Community model (CDC 2015):

1. Each student enters school healthy and then learns about and practices a healthy lifestyle.
2. Each student learns in an environment that is physically and emotionally safe for students and adults.
3. Each student is actively engaged in learning and is connected to the school and broader community.
4. Each student has access to personalized learning and is supported by qualified, caring adults.
5. Each student is challenged academically and prepared for success in college or further study and for employment and participation in a global environment.

Idea 2: Focus on What Is Important

The main purpose of health education is to enable an individual to make informed decisions and to take appropriate actions that affect their own well-being and the well-being of society and the environment.

Idea 3: Focus on the Primary Outcomes of the Curriculum Recommended by the CDC

The CDC (2018) describes less effective health education curricula as those that overemphasize teaching scientific facts and increasing student knowledge. The CDC (2018) suggests that a health education curriculum should emphasize four primary outcomes:

1. Teach functional health information.
2. Shape personal values and beliefs that support healthy behaviors.
3. Shape group norms that value a healthy lifestyle.
4. Develop the essential health skills necessary to adopt, practice, and maintain health-enhancing behaviors.

Idea 4: Increase Understanding Across the Curriculum

A health education curriculum should feature a clear progression toward the goals of preK-12 health education using the big ideas of health education and enduring understandings of the content that are critical for students.

Idea 5: Increase Understanding Systematically

The progression of big ideas should be systematic and should result in deeper understanding of health education as students progress through the curriculum.

Idea 6: Tailor Learning Experiences to Increase Understanding

Learning experiences should reflect the application of health knowledge, informed judgment, and skills that are explicit and consistent with current scientific and educational practice.

Idea 7: Align Professional Development to the Needs of Health Educators

The initial training and later professional development of teachers should be consistent with the teaching and learning methods required to achieve the goals set out in big ideas one and three.

Idea 8: Assessment Matters

Assessment has a key role in health education. The formative assessment of students' learning and the summative assessment must demonstrate student understanding of the content of health education.

Idea 9: Focus on the Whole Child

In working toward these big ideas of health education, school health education programs view learning beyond traditional academic achievement to a model that incorporates a broader view of the skills and knowledge that all children must develop for long-term success. This focus must also include addressing socioemotional learning.

Idea 10: Start Where the Student Is

Teachers must understand who their students are, personalize students' learning, and view students' readiness in terms of both class and individual contexts (see figure 1.1).

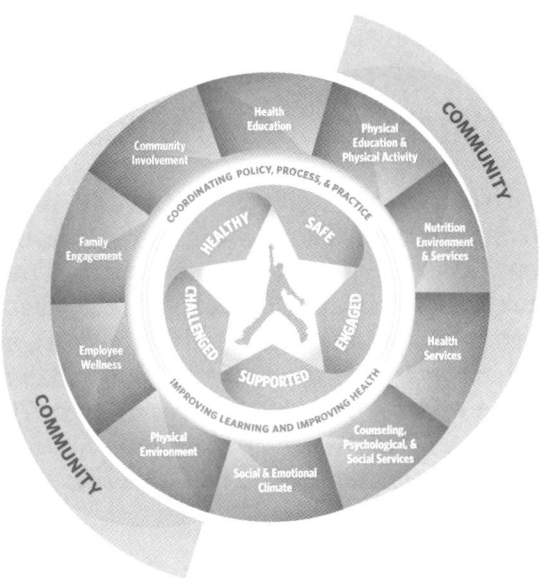

FIGURE 1.1   The Whole School, Whole Child, Whole Community model.

Reprinted from ASCD, Whole School, Whole Community, Whole Child: A Collaborative Approach to Learning and Health (2014).

Our 10 big ideas are grounded in scientific research; in contemporary pedagogical practices recommended by professional associations such as the Association for Supervision and Curriculum Development and SHAPE America; and in public health policy such as the Whole School, Whole Child, Whole Community model and the Centers for Disease Control and Prevention guidelines for health curricula. All of these are critically relevant to teaching health education in preK-12 schools. They are also reflective of the practice-based teacher education movement.

Practice-Based Teacher Education

The practice-based teacher education movement calls for preservice teacher education and for the professional development of practicing teachers. This movement focuses on the work of teaching rather than on things that are tangential to teaching and seeks to give teachers the tools they need for the real world of teaching.

Practice-based teacher education recognizes the complex, relational, and contextual dimensions of teaching discussed at the beginning of this chapter, and it acknowledges that teaching has a professional knowledge base and a set of professional skills that are adapted in different settings according to the needs of students (McDonald et al. 2013). Among the important professional knowledge and skills that teachers need are core teaching practices that result in the most student learning (Forzani 2014).

What Are Core Practices?

Core practices (Grossman et al. 2009), also called high-leverage practices (Ball et al., 2009) or ambitious teaching practices (Windschitl et al. 2018), represent the core task domains of teaching such as using big ideas or designing a sequence of lessons to meet an objective. There are core practices in elementary mathematics (Ball et al. 2009), general teaching practice (Schneider Kavanagh et al. 2017), history (Fogo 2014), music (Millican and Helweh-Forrester 2018), science (Kloser 2014), and special education (McLeskey and Brownell 2015). Core practices typically meet six defining criteria (Grossman et al. 2009, p. 277):

1. Practices that occur with high frequency in teaching
2. Practices that teachers can enact in classrooms across different curricula or instructional approaches
3. Practices that teachers can actually begin to master
4. Practices that allow teachers to learn more about students and about teaching
5. Practices that preserve the integrity and complexity of teaching
6. Practices that are research based and have the potential to improve student achievement

Components of Professional Judgment

A critical feature of teaching is the ability of teachers to adapt instruction and content to address student needs. Remember that an important characteristic of core practices is that teachers can learn from their use. But this learning doesn't happen by chance. It requires that two components of professional judgment, knowledge and reflection, are used. As teachers use their knowledge to plan, enact, and then reflect on their teaching, they are able to learn from their use of these core practices. The use of a core practice requires the teacher's understanding of its nuances and then tinkering with the core practice to adapt to the needs of the student.

Core Practices for Teaching Health Education

Our purpose in writing this book is to provide preservice teachers, in-service teachers, and teacher educators with the core practices of teaching health education. Our goals are to

1. provide explanation and rationale for core practices of teaching health education,

2. situate these core practices of teaching health education within the practice-based teacher education movement,

3. provide clear guidance on how to use these core practices in health classrooms, and

4. support teacher efforts in using core practices of teaching health education to address the big ideas in health education.

Our choices for core practices are based on our collective experiences as health teacher educators and the extensive pedagogical literature in support of core practices (Ball et al. 2009; Fogo 2014; Grossman et al. 2009; Kloser 2014; Millican and Helweh-Forrester 2018; Schneider Kavanagh et al. 2017; Windschitl et al. 2018).

We have organized core practices of teaching health education into three parts. The first focuses on planning the health education curriculum. The second part discusses the pedagogy of health education. The third part addresses practices that help teachers to reflect and grow across their careers. Figure 1.2 shows the organization of the three parts and their core practices.

Each chapter introduces a core practice for health education and includes a vignette that illustrates the use of the core practice. We then provide an explanation and rationale for and examples of the core practices. Finally, we provide clear guidance on how to use each core

Part 1 Planning for the teaching of content of health education	**Part 2** Pedagogy for health education	**Part 3** Growing as a teacher
• Teaching with big ideas • Enduring ideas • Essential questions • Sequencing content • Representing content to students • Assessing learning	• Organizational routines/procedure rules and expectations • Building a classroom community that is safe, caring, and focused on learning • Facilitating classroom discussion • Providing feedback to students • Adapting instruction to meet the needs of students • Developing decision-making skills in students	• Reflecting on teaching • Reflecting on lesson improvement

FIGURE 1.2   Core practices for teaching health education

practice in health classrooms. *Core Teaching Practices for Health Education* can be used as a pedagogical guide for teacher educators, as a supporting pedagogical resource in health education methods classes or for practicing teachers, or as a stand-alone resource in student teaching for preservice teachers.

Summary

The chapters that follow address teaching practices seldom discussed in depth in health education but that are commonplace in other subject areas. Using the teaching practices found in this book will make you a better teacher because they will build on your existing knowledge. You can have confidence that these practices are grounded not only in a strong rationale but also with strong research evidence (Hattie 2009; Marzano et al. 2003). Our goal is to improve teaching effectiveness and student learning in health education. Health education has suffered from a lack of focus on pedagogical teaching skills. Moreover, the field has been disconnected from teacher education occurring in other subjects. The big ideas in this chapter represent important considerations for health educators and teacher educators in improving the teaching of health education in schools. Importantly, teachers using the core practices in this book not only are using effective teaching practices, but they can adapt them in different classes and across their careers.

CHAPTER 2

Big Ideas

Imagine a group of middle school students in class engaging in a lesson on decision-making. The teacher, Ms. Cacho, has worksheets, a PowerPoint presentation, and a series of activities for the students to use to demonstrate their understanding of the lesson. As a concluding activity, the students are asked to take a short quiz followed by a class discussion of the quiz answers. After class Ms. Cacho reviews the quizzes and reflects on the discussion. It is clear to her that the students know pieces of the lesson, but for the most part they are not making connections between the content, nor do they see the content as relevant to their lives.

Ms. Cacho decides to revisit the lesson in the next class and to reorganize the future lessons in the unit differently. She organizes the unit around one big idea: Healthy choices influence our physical, mental, and emotional well-being. She next determines the enduring understandings related to this big idea that she wants her students to retain. Enduring understandings, explained further in chapter 3, frame the big ideas that give meaning and lasting importance to essential curriculum elements. She chooses three enduring understandings for this unit at this grade level: (1) making good health decisions requires the ability to access and evaluate reliable resources, (2) the decisions we make affect our lives, and (3) informed decision-making is empowering.

Ms. Cacho then organizes the unit around four essential questions around which she will focus the lesson content and activities. Students connect to enduring understandings and big ideas through essential questions, which are discussed in chapter 4. Essential questions are central to the study of health education curricula, and their use promotes inquiry and unpacking of health education. Ms. Cacho's essential questions are these: (1) How should you judge the quality of health information? (2) How should you make sense of conflicting health information? (3) How do the decisions you make now affect your lives, now and later? (4) What does it mean to say you are in control? After each lesson Ms. Cacho reviews her assessments and concludes that she has good evidence that her students understood the big idea, demonstrated that they could connect the understandings they examined in the lessons to the big idea, and were able to apply these understandings to their own lives.

Many subject area experts in other disciplines (e.g., math, history, and science), school districts, and teacher education programs use big ideas as a key pedagogical principle (Wiggens 2010; Windschitl et al., 2018). Big ideas allow teachers to

- respond to students' need to gain a coherent perspective of a subject area's content,
- provide a framework for instructional activities to help students understand the content,
- use a rationale in the selection of the relevant curriculum content in a subject area, and
- develop a curriculum built on the progression of a subject area's big ideas.

What Is a Big Idea?

A big idea is a concise statement of a health outcome. It is a way to package all the lesson's pieces of knowledge and experiences together so that students can see them as related. The notion is similar to seeing the picture of a puzzle as you start to put the pieces together. That picture guides the organization of the puzzle pieces. Wiggins (2010, p. 1) calls an idea big "if it helps us make sense of lots of confusing experiences and seemingly isolated facts." Big ideas connect knowledge with experiences learned in a unit. Here are five examples of big ideas in health:

- Understanding that we are all both similar and different helps us communicate well.
- Taking responsibility for one's own health is an essential step toward developing and maintaining a healthy lifestyle.
- Sexuality is a natural and healthy part of living.
- Knowing about our bodies and making choices helps us look after ourselves.
- Healthy relationships can help us lead rewarding and fulfilling lives.

In the introductory vignette, "Healthy choices influence our physical, mental, and emotional well-being" was the big idea. Ms. Cacho used that big idea to organize the enduring understandings and the essential questions of the unit's content to meet her state standard: "Students will demonstrate the ability to use decision-making skills to enhance health." Figure 2.1 shows the interrelationships of a standard, big ideas, enduring understandings, and essential questions. Big ideas are driven by standards that students are expected to meet and are operationalized through the use of enduring understandings and essential questions.

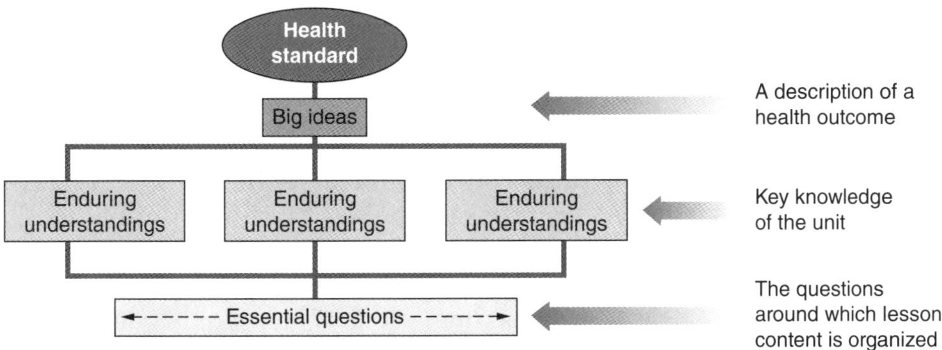

FIGURE 2.1   Interrelationships of a standard, big ideas, enduring understandings, and essential questions.

For teachers, organizing teaching around a small number of big ideas is an efficient and effective strategy. Big ideas organize content to create an understanding of the connectivity of health education across the curriculum and grade levels. Such understanding in turn allows teachers to make use of connections and concepts within and between big ideas.

For students, big ideas create coherence by organizing and connecting ideas. A big idea might be stated differently by teachers. For example, one teacher might say, "You are the decision maker," and another might frame it as, "Health is personal power." Regardless of the phrasing, the meaning is the same. Big ideas occur across grade levels (e.g., preK-12), stand the test of time (e.g., contagious diseases), are applied across different subject areas (e.g., implicit bias), recur in a variety of content (e.g., being a decision maker is relevant in a variety of health content areas), and are applied to contexts that students may not yet have encountered in their lives (e.g., reflection) (Wiggins 2010).

Big Ideas Across the Curriculum

Big ideas have been used in two ways across curricula. One way is to use the same set of big ideas, which are unpacked in more depth with each successive grade level. For example, Roosevelt Public School in New Jersey uses four big ideas across their K-6 curriculum:

- Taking responsibility for one's own health is an essential step toward developing and maintaining a healthy lifestyle.
- Critical thinking, decision-making, problem-solving, leadership, and communication skills are essential to making informed personal, family, and community health decisions.

- Knowledge about drugs and medicines informs decision-making related to personal wellness and the wellness of others.
- Understanding the various aspects of human relationships and sexuality assists in making good choices about healthy living.

A second way to use big ideas is to expand on them with increasingly sophisticated description. For example, table 2.1 shows the big ideas used in health education from kindergarten to year 12 in the health curriculum. Although this example shows four big ideas per grade level, the columns should not be viewed as thematic development because these big ideas grow to encompass some elements of earlier ideas. In short, some big ideas overlap over time. However, a curriculum could use big ideas that intentionally remain the same over time.

TABLE 2.1   Big Ideas in Health Education Across the Curriculum

Grade level	BIG IDEAS		
Kindergarten	Knowing about myself and others helps me understand myself and others, which helps us build healthy relationships.	Knowing about my body helps me look after myself.	Good health is composed of physical, mental, social, and emotional well-being.
Grade 3	Using healthy behaviors and being safe protects me and others.	Communicating and managing my emotions enable me to develop and maintain healthy relationships.	The elements of physical, emotional, social, and mental health are interconnected.
Grade 5	Having healthy relationships helps me be connected.	Understanding the various aspects of health helps me to develop a balanced lifestyle.	My personal choices, my social interactions, and environmental factors influence my health and well-being.
Grade 7	Learning about the similarities and differences in others helps me understand my community.	Change is constant in our lives.	The choices we make influence our physical, mental, social, and emotional well-being.
Grade 9	Advocating for the health and well-being of others is a moral responsibility.	Healthy relationships are necessary for our growth as human beings.	The choices we make influence our physical, mental, social, and emotional well-being.

Based on BC's Curriculum, *Physical and Health Education K*.

Choosing Big Ideas

How do you determine what big ideas to use? An important factor is whether this is a district activity, a group of teachers engaging in their own professional development for planning health, or a solo endeavor. Though choosing big ideas can be done alone, it is best done with other health educators for strength and ease in numbers. If this is done at a district level, you are probably working on developing a preK-12 framework. If you are working within specific grade levels, your focus will be on the grades you teach. A critical question that needs to be determined across grades, whether it is preK-12 or a small set of grades, is whether the wording of the big ideas will change over time, as shown in table 2.1, or whether you will stick with the same, as Roosevelt Public Schools decided to do with their K-6 curriculum.

Big ideas should be a generative topic, not a theme. Themes are smaller units of understanding often used to apply skills. In contrast, generative topics have three elements: (1) centrality to the discipline, (2) richness of linking, and (3) relevance to students. Generative topics help teachers look for transferability and acceptability of ideas from different perspectives. Big ideas should be phrased as a sentence with a verb that provides direction and ideas for teachers and learners to explore the idea (Mitchell et al. 2017).

We suggest two steps to determine big ideas.

Step 1: Choose Your Topic

Teachers should use their professional judgment to select big ideas, using curriculum guides, health standards, and textbooks as guides. This task can be performed in many ways, including creating an outline on the computer or on a chalkboard or whiteboard, but we recommend index cards or sticky notes. Begin with one standard, and then write one potential big idea per card. At this stage don't worry about the exact wording; that will change. Just get your big ideas down until you have four or five. On each card write the standard that the big idea represents. Next repeat this with the remaining standards, doing one standard at a time. It is appropriate to reuse big ideas across standards, but be sure to write it on a new card.

Step 2: Organize Your Ideas

Set all the cards out on a table or sticky notes on the wall, and arrange them in columns by standard. Align the cards to show the relationships of the big ideas to each other. Your goal is to reduce by consolidating the big ideas within a standard. Reduction occurs whenever you place a card under an existing big idea and work on the wording. As you repeat this activity with each standard, your goal is to reduce not only by consolidating the big ideas within each standard but also by consolidating across standards. In a typical curriculum that uses the same big ideas for each grade level, you should aim to create no more than four big ideas. To get to this point, keep placing cards under other cards, rewording the big idea in the process.

Summary

Big ideas are hugely beneficial in organizing the content in the health education curriculum. They create greater opportunity for generative instruction tied to student values and interests. The result is deeper, more connected understandings. Developing big ideas is a process, not a destination. Big ideas are intended to change over time so that they can be refined and elaborated upon. In this chapter we have provided a strategy for the development of big ideas. It is not the only way to develop a big idea, but it is the best way we have used. Creating big ideas requires time and knowledge of the health curriculum and standards. For that reason, we recommend that big ideas are developed in collaboration with other teachers rather than alone. The remaining chapters of this cluster pull from the use of big ideas. We believe that big ideas will ultimately make teaching health education easier than the process often used in classrooms today.

CHAPTER 3

Using Enduring Understandings to Focus Student Learning

In chapter 2, we introduced readers to Ms. Cacho, who was struggling with how to make sense of and organize the large amount of health education content in health education. Ms. Cacho worked hard to identify the big ideas derived from the health education standards in her state. As noted in chapter 2, a big idea is a way to package all the pieces of knowledge and experiences in the instructional unit together in such a way that students see them as related. To describe a big idea, we used the metaphor of seeing a picture of a puzzle before putting the pieces of the puzzle together. In this chapter we look at the pieces of the puzzle. When you put a puzzle together, you look for the pieces' similarities such as color and shape and then match those to the picture of the puzzle. For example, when working on a puzzle that is a picture of a forest scene, you might look for blue pieces for the sky or green pieces for the trees. Similarly, when looking at health education content, we use enduring understandings as the pieces of the big idea. It is the teacher's task to look for the common elements of the content relative to the big idea. This chapter helps you do that. As a reminder, enduring understandings are situated between big ideas (see chapter 2) and essential questions (see chapter 4), as depicted in figure 3.1.

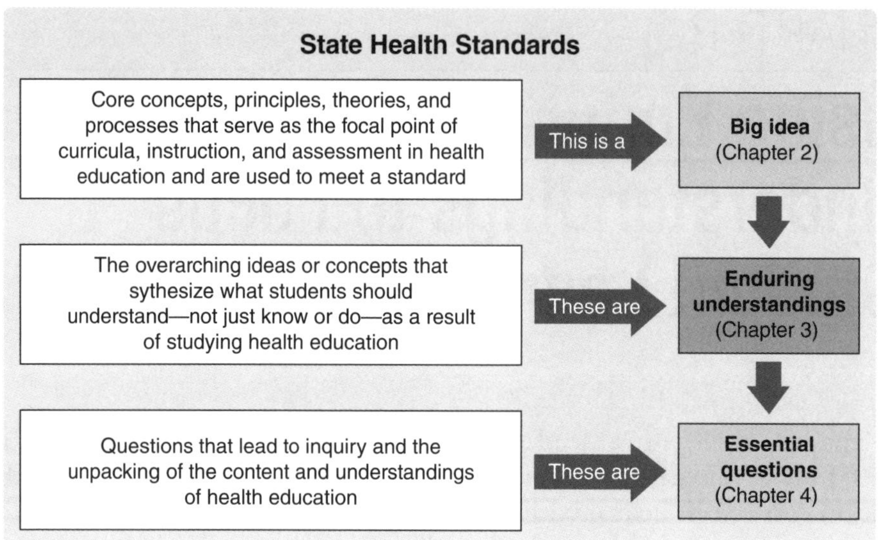

FIGURE 3.1 Big ideas, enduring understandings, and essential questions.

What Are Enduring Understandings?

Enduring understandings are overarching ideas or concepts related to the big idea. They synthesize what students should understand—not just know or do—as a result of health education. Such understandings are interpretive and therefore nuanced relative to a setting. For example, consider this enduring understanding: "Recognizing risk factors and using risk-reducing strategies can prevent health consequences." Consider the issue of social distancing and the wearing of masks during the COVID-19 pandemic. If people from separate households do not wear masks while speaking to each other, the implementation of this enduring understanding would call for greater social distance than if they were wearing masks.

Characteristics of Enduring Understandings

Enduring understandings display the following characteristics. First, enduring understandings provide a conceptual foundation or framework for studying health education. Consider this understanding: Mental and emotional health affects a person's physical health and overall well-being. This understanding provides a framework for informed decision-making relative to mental and emotional health.

Second, enduring understandings are transferable beyond health education. The earlier example of COVID-19 displays recognizing risk factors based on the setting and other people and determining which risk-reduction strategy to use. This is like learning to drive a car in different road conditions, which requires making a series of judgments: which lane to be in, what speed to be driving at, the distance between your car and the next. Ultimately, you cannot teach a person all the possible road conditions or circumstances for COVID-19, but you can teach adaptability and analysis of context.

Third, enduring understandings often recur throughout lessons. The examples of COVID-19 and driving not only should recur throughout lessons in the same unit but throughout units of different content. For example, the enduring understanding of risk reduction should recur in units on communicable disease, body systems, analyzing influences, and decision-making.

Finally, enduring understandings are ideas or concepts that students should revisit over the course of their lifetimes as they make decisions relative to their health. If students understand risk reduction, they can revisit it in physical activity and self-management units, and even when they have graduated and are making decisions about going to the doctor or buying a new piece of hiking equipment. An enduring understanding lays the health foundation for the rest of students' lives.

Examples of Health Education Enduring Understandings

Enduring understandings are typically framed as declarative sentences that present major curriculum generalizations and recurrent ideas. A declarative sentence is a statement that tells us something or gives information. The following list shows some examples of enduring understandings from Wallingford Public Schools in Connecticut.

- Personal choices impact current and long-term outcomes on individuals, family, and society.
- Mental and emotional health affects a person's physical health and overall well-being.
- Assertive communication skills enhance health by avoiding or reducing health risks.
- Accessing and evaluating health information, products, and services will improve a person's ability to make healthy decisions and one's quality of life.
- Recognizing risk factors and applying risk-reducing strategies can prevent negative health consequences.
- Individuals need to express their sexuality in ways that are both healthy and responsible.
- Understanding puberty helps to facilitate the emotional transition from childhood to adolescence.

- Everyone has special and unique qualities.
- Individuals embrace diversity as contributing members of a larger community.

Reprinted by permission from Wallinford Public Schools. https://www.wallingford.k12.ct.us/uploaded/Curriculum/PE_AND_HEALTH_K-12/Health_K-12_Enduring_Und_and_Essential_Questions.pdf

Table 3.1 presents enduring understandings from Maryland State Health Education Standards that are developed across grade levels.

TABLE 3.1 Enduring Understandings Relative to Maryland State Health Education Standards Developed Across Grade Levels

Unit and standard	Grade 6	Grade 7	Grade 8	Grade 10
Mental and Emotional Health Standard 1—Students will demonstrate the ability to use mental and emotional health knowledge, skills, and strategies to enhance their self-concept and their relationship with others.	Lifelong personal well-being is achieved through **choices and decisions** based on healthy attitudes and behaviors.	Lifelong personal well-being is achieved through **effective communication and decisions** based on healthy attitudes and behaviors.	Lifelong personal well-being is achieved through **effective communication and decisions** based on healthy attitudes and behaviors.	Lifelong personal well-being is achieved through **motivation** and **commitment** to maintain healthy attitudes and behaviors.
Alcohol, Tobacco, and Other Drugs Standard 2—Students will demonstrate the ability to use drug knowledge, decision-making skills, and health-enhancing strategies to address the nonuse, use, and abuse of medication, alcohol, tobacco, and other drugs.	The **decision not to misuse** alcohol, tobacco, and other drugs is essential to lifelong wellness.	The **decision not to misuse** alcohol, tobacco, and other drugs is essential to lifelong wellness.	**Health literacy and resistance skills** are essential to healthy choices promoting lifelong wellness.	**Health literacy and resistance skills** are essential to healthy choices promoting lifelong wellness.

Reprinted from Maryland Public Schools (Rockville, Maryland).

How to Determine and Write Enduring Understandings

There are two types of enduring understandings: overarching and topical. *Overarching enduring understandings* are transferable and occur in multiple units of study in health education. An example of an overarching understanding follows: "Assertive communication skills enhance health by avoiding and/or reducing health risks." This example can be used to address most health education content areas. Overarching enduring understandings also explain to students why they have to learn something. *Topical enduring understandings* are specific ideas within a unit that students should grasp. An example of a topical enduring understanding follows: "Sex hormones impact decision-making of males and females differently." In this example, the enduring understanding is only related to sex education, but it has enduring meaning for students. However, it can be used and expanded upon across grade levels.

We suggest that you base your unit design on enduring understandings that you intend for students to gain. There is no correct ratio of overarching to topical enduring understandings, nor is there a number of enduring understandings that is desired, though most health education units typically have three to five.

Writing enduring understandings requires that you use your content knowledge and familiarity with standards, benchmarks, and performance indicators. In planning enduring understandings, ask yourself two questions: (1) What long-term concepts should students understand from this unit? (2) What do I want my students to understand that will allow them to learn as they use the enduring understandings? These questions drive your formulation of enduring understandings that are the core of the health education unit.

Checklist for Writing Enduring Understandings

Enduring understandings should follow these rules:

- Written as a complete sentence
- Written in the present tense
- Connect two concepts using a verb
- Reference key understandings in the unit
- Apply to other units (overarching) or specifically to this unit (topical)
- Transferable across grade levels

Enduring understandings should be complete sentences in the present tense, and are a sandwich of a concept-verb-concept describing the relation between two concepts. For example, "communication [concept] enhances [verb] health [concept]," or "sex hormones [concept] impact [verb] decisions [concept]." Begin with "Students understand that," and complete the sentence using two or more concepts from your standards or unit of study. Look for the two concepts and the verb in the following examples. The concepts are boldfaced, and the verbs are underlined.

- **Accessing and evaluating health information, products, and services** <u>will improve</u> **a person's ability to make healthy decisions and one's quality of life.**
- **Recognizing risk factors and applying risk-reducing strategies** <u>can prevent</u> **health consequences.**
- **Individuals** <u>should express</u> **their sexuality in ways that are both healthy and responsible.**
- **Understanding puberty** <u>helps</u> **to facilitate the emotional transition from childhood to adolescence.**

Be sure to write enduring understandings in age- and developmentally appropriate language so that all your students can know what they will be learning.

Figure 3.2 presents the standard Ms. Cacho is addressing and the interrelationships of the standard, big idea, and enduring questions.

As Ms. Cacho explores her enduring understandings, she notices a number of things. First, writing enduring understanding gets easier the more familiar she is with the content and the standards. Second, over time she is able to refine her enduring understandings. Third, discussing and developing enduring understandings with other health educators, either within a formal curriculum or as peers, is a valuable exercise. Finally, Ms. Cacho realizes that health education content is more manageable now that she is aligned with the standards, big ideas, and enduring understandings. However, she wonders how to teach enduring understandings to her students. In chapter 4, we will explore this and essential questions.

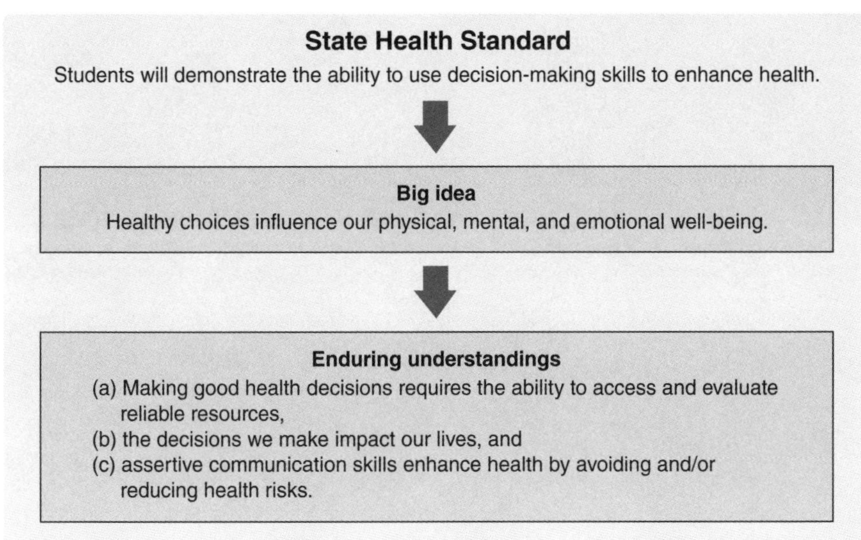

FIGURE 3.2　The interrelationship of Ms. Cacho's standard, big idea, and enduring understandings.

Summary

Enduring understandings are overarching ideas or concepts related to a big idea. Using enduring understandings helps teachers to plan more effectively and efficiently because they capture the big picture of a unit without getting mired in each individual standard. Using enduring understandings allows teachers to systematically and gradually deepen an understanding of the content of health education as students advance through a curriculum. Enduring understandings helps students make sense of the enormous content in health education. They allow students to see the shape of the forest, not just the individual trees. This kind of understanding is a degree of sophistication in teaching health education that is typically not present when the curriculum is viewed as a set of unrelated instructional units.

CHAPTER 4

Using Essential Questions to Promote Enduring Understandings

When we finished chapter 3, Ms. Cacho was wondering how to teach enduring understandings to her students. Typically, when Ms. Cacho teaches her class, she asks most of her questions in such a way that students can provide specific answers relative to the lesson content. She sometimes asks questions to frame the content she is about to teach, but these questions are typically tied to the lesson and are therefore focused in scope. In this chapter we describe the use of *essential questions*. Figure 4.1 depicts how essential questions come after the big ideas and enduring understandings are determined.

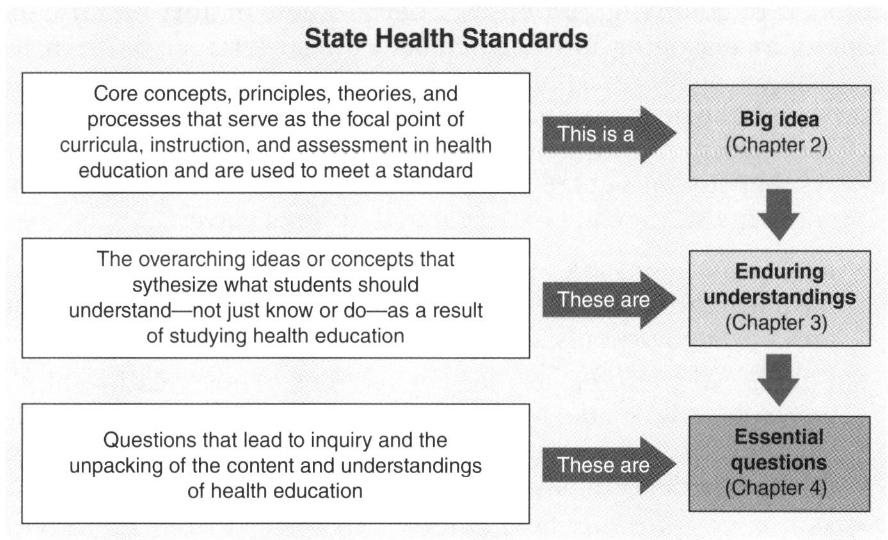

FIGURE 4.1 Essential questions are situated after big ideas and enduring understandings.

Essential questions are aligned with enduring understandings, which in turn are derived from the big ideas. It is through these questions that students unpack the subject matter of health education and find meaning. The big ideas serve to define the core concepts, principles, theories, and processes of health education relative to the standards; enduring understandings describe what students should understand; and essential questions frame how the big ideas and enduring understandings are represented to the students (Wiggins and McTighe 1998). To use the puzzle metaphor described in chapters 2 and 3, the big idea is the picture of the puzzle to which you refer when assembling it. Enduring understandings are the puzzle pieces. Essential questions are what you would ask to determine if the pieces fit together (e.g., How can I determine if this blue matches the sky or the water in the picture?).

What Are Essential Questions?

Essential questions are used by teachers to focus the lesson content. A question is essential if it can be asked throughout our lifetimes; links to core ideas in health education (i.e., big ideas and enduring understandings); and is phrased in a way that prompts students to inquire and make sense of important, complex ideas. Essential questions cannot be answered with a yes or no or in one sentence, because they often require a rationale or qualifying responses. They promote inquiry because they often require reasoning and research before an answer can be given, and even then, the answer may be conditional. Essential questions are used to show both the nuance of particular viewpoints and the application of health education in a student's daily life, and they ultimately represent the ways that students come to understand health education content.

Essential questions can be categorized in three ways:

- *Factual questions* ask for facts that can be researched and typically have a right or wrong answer. Example: How do you determine appropriate portion sizes?

- *Conceptual questions* ask for connections to and relationships of concepts to be made, leading students to a higher level of understanding. Example: How can communication enhance my personal health and develop positive relationships?

- *Debatable questions* lead students to offer various viewpoints. Example: How can goal setting enhance and improve my health?

Characteristics of Essential Questions

Essential questions

- can be asked throughout our lifetimes;
- link to core ideas in health education (i.e., big ideas and enduring understandings);
- are phrased in ways that prompt students to inquire and make sense of important, complex ideas;
- are used by teachers to focus the lesson content;
- promote inquiry; and
- unpack the content to show both the nuance of particular viewpoints and the application of health education in a student's daily life.

Examples of Health Education Essential Questions Related to Enduring Understandings

Table 4.1 shows enduring understandings and essential questions related to how Wallingford Public Schools in Connecticut used their health curriculum. Both the enduring understandings and the essential questions can be used across a variety of instructional units. This is why enduring understandings and essential questions should be created as a curriculum, not just as a unit.

TABLE 4.1   Enduring Understandings and Essential Questions

Enduring understandings	Essential questions
• Personal choices impact current and long-term outcomes on individuals, family and society. • Mental and emotional health affects a person's physical health and overall well-being. • Assertive communication skills enhance health by avoiding or reducing health risks. • Accessing and evaluating health information, products, and services will improve a person's ability to make healthy decisions and one's quality of life. • Recognizing risk factors and applying risk-reducing strategies can prevent health consequences.	• How and where can I locate health resources? • What can I do to avoid or reduce health risks? • What influences my behaviors and decisions? • How can assertive communication skills help me to develop a healthy lifestyle? • What do I need to know to make good decisions and stay healthy? • How can I make good decisions and stay healthy? • How can goal setting enhance and improve my health? • How can I promote accurate health information and behavior for myself and others?

(continued)

Table 4.1   *(continued)*

Enduring understandings	Essential questions
• Individuals need to express their sexuality in ways that are both healthy and responsible. • Understanding puberty helps to facilitate the emotional transition from childhood to adolescence. • Everyone has special and unique qualities. • Individuals embrace diversity as contributing members of a larger community.	• How and where can I seek help? • How does my behavior reflect my personal choices? • What can I do to prevent and resolve conflict? • How can communication enhance my personal health and develop positive relationships? • How do a person's unique talents contribute to a larger community?

Reprinted from Maryland Public Schools (Rockville, Maryland).

Ms. Cacho wrote four essential questions: (1) How should you judge the quality of health information? (2) How should you make sense of conflicting health information? (3) How do the decisions we make now impact our lives, now and later? (4) What does it mean to say you are in control? Figure 4.2 shows the interrelationship of the standard, big idea, enduring understandings, and essential questions that she chose.

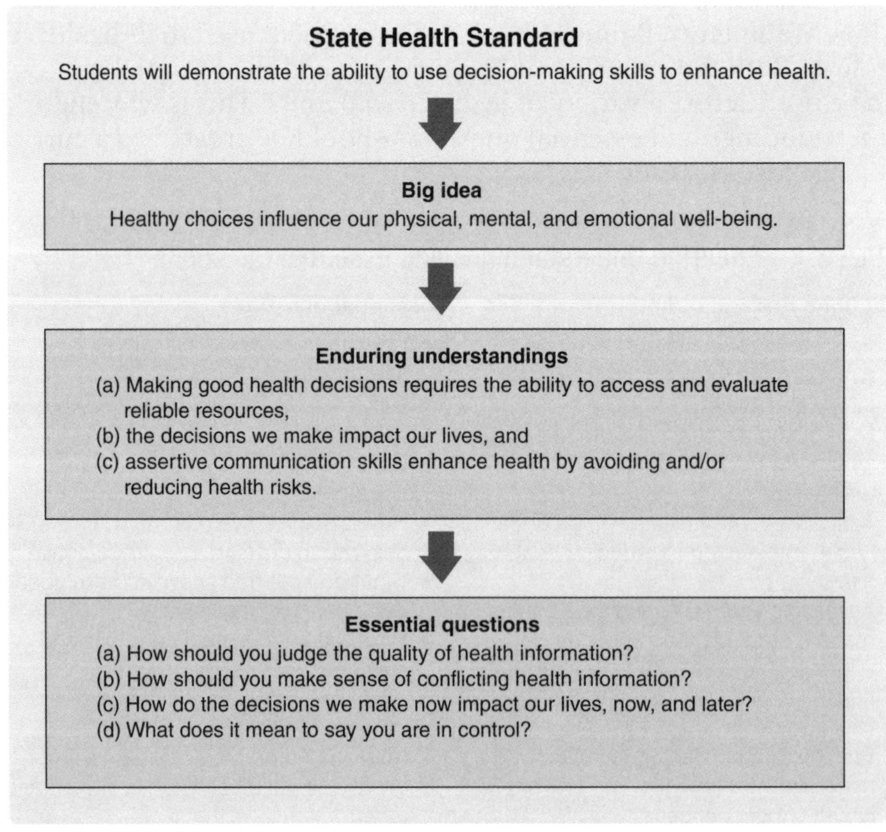

FIGURE 4.2   An example of a big idea and its enduring understandings and essential questions.

How to Write Essential Questions

In writing your essential questions, keep in mind the following:

1. Although there is no set number for how many questions you should create, it is helpful to aim for one or two per lesson, or three to five per unit of study.
2. Write your questions in age-appropriate language. The questions are for your students, not another teacher, to answer.
3. Essential questions should be one sentence and short.
4. Make the questions engaging and thought-provoking.
5. The questions should tie specifically to your enduring understandings.
6. Design questions that reflect the standards and big ideas of your content area.
7. Write essential questions starting with the words or phrases *How*, *Why*, *If*, or *What impact*.
8. Sequence your questions so that they lead logically from one to another.
9. If a question is too specific or could be answered with a few words or a sentence, it is not an essential question.
10. The question should not have one right answer. It may have many.

Summary

At this point in unit and curriculum design, both the forest and the trees should be visible, and the interrelationships of standards, big ideas, enduring understandings, and essential questions should be very clear. Ms. Cacho, like many teachers at this point, feels a sense of relief that the amorphous content of health education is manageable and that the messages she wants students to take with them beyond the school and throughout life are clearly articulated. In the next chapters we will discuss how to sequence content and activities in health education and how to assess the content.

CHAPTER 5

Sequencing Health Content

Ms. Zeinz is teaching new content in her mental health unit to her class of eighth graders, whom she has taught for their previous two years of middle school. During her first class she connects the content to the prior knowledge of the students, much of which she has taught to them already. Her hopes for the lesson dwindle, however, as the students respond in ways that lead her to conclude that she needs to start from scratch and cover material that she thought she had previously covered. Most frustrating to her is that the conceptual understandings that she has worked so hard to develop in the past appear to have not been retained by her students. At lunch Ms. Zeinz shares her frustration with her friend Mr. Li, a math teacher, who commented, "I totally understand. I just gave my class a test to determine what they had learned last year, and the results were very disappointing. It was as if I didn't teach much of the content." They both groan in frustration. After school that day, Ms. Zeinz stays to completely rewrite her unit. One consequence of this is that she will not have the time to go as deeply into the content as she would like.

What Ms. Zeinz and Mr. Li are describing is the students' lack of retention of the previous content. One reason for this is that too often concepts and knowledge are taught in ways that are disjointed and disconnected from each other and from classroom experiences. Some years ago a Chinese researcher studying in the United States compared the teaching of basic math in elementary schools in each country (Ma 1999). She discovered that many teachers in the United States taught the content and then moved on with little recurring reference to previous content. In contrast, the Chinese teachers she studied spent considerable time revisiting previously taught content as they introduced new content. In short, their students encountered the same content frequently throughout their schooling. In this chapter we present two ways to think about sequencing health content: the spiral curriculum and learning progressions. Both are practical ways to improve student retention and understanding of the subject matter and to avoid teacher frustration with poor student retention of previous content. In this chapter and throughout the book the term *content* refers to the content of health education that is taught to students in K-12 settings.

The Spiral Curriculum

The spiral curriculum (Bruner 1960) is a curriculum design in which content or big ideas (see chapter 2) and enduring understandings (see chapter 3) are revisited repeatedly throughout the curriculum. However, previously taught big ideas or enduring understandings are not repeated, but students are presented with deepening layers of complexity or applications that serve to strengthen and expand understanding of a topic. Figure 5.1 of a spiral curriculum demonstrates recurring big ideas, which are represented by the shaded parts of the ribbon that are progressively introduced across grade levels with increasing depth.

A spiral curriculum displays the following features:

- Content, big ideas, and enduring understandings are revisited within and across grades.

- Content, big ideas, and enduring understandings are intentionally expanded in their complexity and nuance. Each return visit is characterized by objectives, activities, and experiences that strengthen and expand student understanding.

- New understandings are related to prior learning. Prior learning serves as a prerequisite for the later learning.

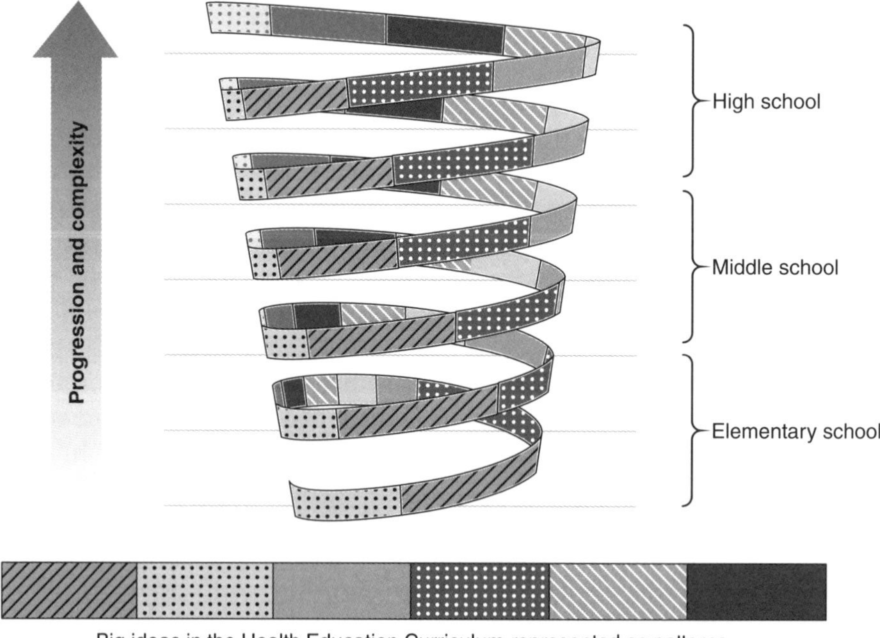

FIGURE 5.1   A spiral curriculum demonstrating recurring big ideas, progressively introduced across grade levels with increasing depth.

The advantages of this approach include:

- Alignment and congruence in student learning within and across grade levels and order to the increasingly complex nature of health education
- Opportunities for the teacher to incrementally introduce content moving from simple to complex by revisiting big ideas or enduring understandings
- Better student understanding by exploring the same health education topics at deepening levels

In figure 5.2 and the sidebar Big Idea: What Is Healthy Eating? we provide an example of a how a big idea—"What is healthy eating?"—is developed across grades. We have used many of the objectives from the health curriculum of Madison Public Schools in Connecticut. The objectives are arranged from earliest introduction to last introduction in the curriculum across grade levels in sequential and incremental ways. Taught in this way, prior knowledge is revisited cyclically and depth is increased across the K-12 curriculum.

How to Construct a Spiral Curriculum in Health Education

First, determine what the students must know and be able to do. We recommend using big ideas (see chapter 2). Next, for each big idea, use either enduring understandings (see chapter 3) or objectives (see figure 5.2) to sequence the understandings across the curriculum. It is helpful to work backwards from your enduring understanding or objective, or final outcome.

Second, once you have established what your students must know and be able to do, develop assessments (see chapter 7) that align strongly with the enduring understandings or objectives that you have used to build the curriculum. Next, select instructional tasks and activities that closely align with the enduring understandings and assessment. This alignment is a prescription for success and differs greatly from the typical content-driven approach to teaching, where the teacher teaches a piece of content that is often disconnected from previous learning.

While creating a spiral curriculum is best done at the district level, teachers can do this themselves for the grade levels they teach in the absence of a district effort. One of the key advantages for teachers is that it provides clarity and direction in their teaching.

Big Idea: What Is Healthy Eating?

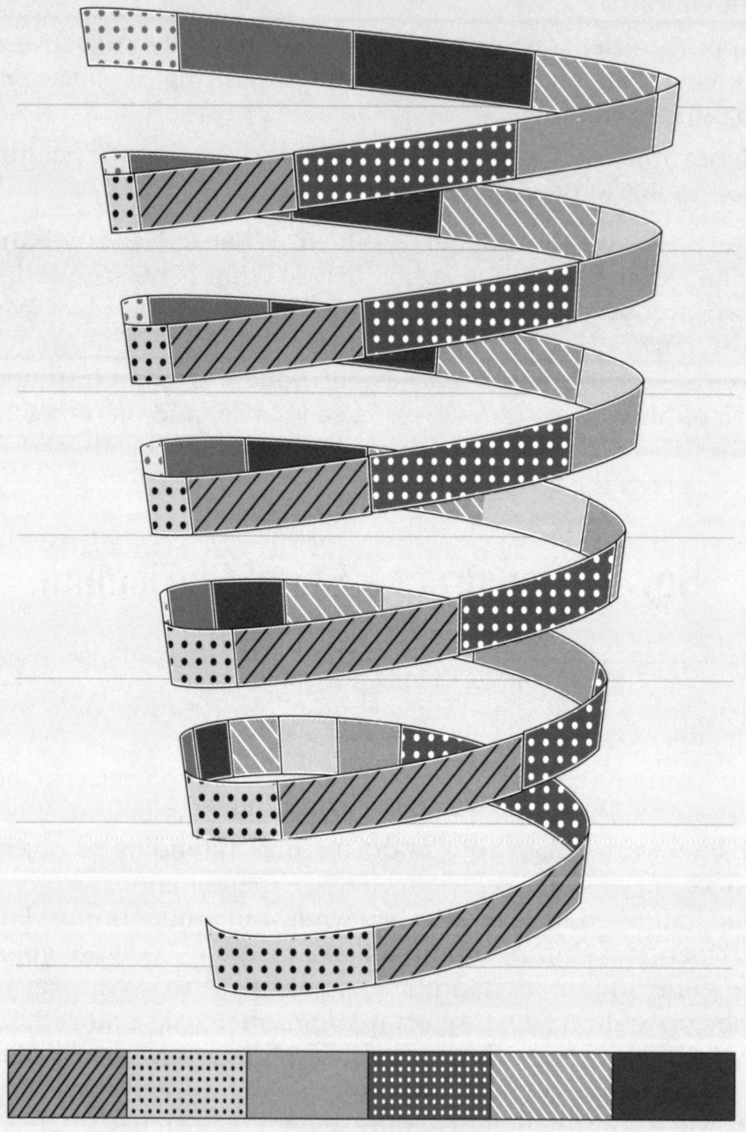

FIGURE 5.2 A spiral curriculum demonstrating the big idea "What is healthy eating?" relative to objectives organized across grade levels.

Grades 9-12 Objectives

- Develop individual diet plans for self and family. Differentiate the diet requirements for different lifestyles.

- Consider the impact of dieting in causing or contributing to specific diseases and health conditions. Assess the influence of economic, social, and emotional factors on personal eating habits.

- Analyze the impact the media have on food selections. List the US dietary guidelines for healthy lifestyles. Assess the impact of economics on food selection.

- Analyze the impact of food sources on world hunger.

Grades 7-8 Objectives

- Evaluate daily food intake in terms of nutritional requirements for adolescents. Analyze the relationship between food intake, physical activity, and body weight. Evaluate temporary and long-term health problems associated with poor eating habits. Analyze reasons for eating (e.g., sustain life, boredom, anxiety, low self-image).

- Recognize and appreciate the nutritional value in cultural and ethnic foods. Weigh the impact of the media on eating lifestyles.

- Be able to assess food labeling and compare costs for nutritional value.

Grades 4-6 Objectives

- Describe social, emotional, ethnic, and cultural influences on attitudes about foods and eating habits.

- Explain the different nutritional needs of individuals depending on age, sex, activity, and state of health.

- Appraise the impact of diet on growth and development during puberty.

- Describe the function of the major nutrients.

- Classify foods on the basis of nutrient content.

Grades K-3 Objectives

- Conclude that a large variety of food is necessary for good health.

- Select foods, based on ethnic and cultural preferences, that promote growth and development.

- Identify foods that are high in fiber, such as fruits and vegetables, whole grains, and legumes.

- Identify foods for breakfast and snacks that provide energy and nutrients for work and play.

- Describe the effect of foods on fitness and growth.

- Illustrate food combinations that provide a balanced daily meal.

Learning Progression

Another way to present health education is to use a learning progression. Learning progressions are defined as "successively more sophisticated ways of thinking about a topic that can follow and build on one another as children learn about a topic over a broad span of time" (National Research Council 2007, p. 217). The sequence of how students come to understand big ideas and content is important. At the heart of a learning progression is a developmental perspective that takes into account that prior knowledge is a prerequisite for future knowledge and that knowledge is best taught and learned incrementally.

A learning progression is a coherent and sequenced set of building blocks that students must learn as prerequisites in order to learn a more distant curricular aim (Popham 2007). Learning progressions describe the sequence of learning in a domain or subject matter of big ideas over many years or just a term's work with a greater degree of specificity. Learning progressions can occur over a relatively short period (e.g., over the course of an instructional unit). To illustrate, consider the sequence of four enduring understandings that represent a learning progression, each enduring understanding building on previous knowledge in ways that broaden the student's understanding and application.

Some learning progressions span the development of understanding across grade levels, while others exist within a grade level. In particular, learning progressions scaffold student understanding. The term *scaffolding* describes how teachers provide and adjust support for learning by intentionally drawing on students' ability to problem-solve by networking with classmates to extend their understanding of a topic. It is like learning a new skill and then being presented with new challenges that you must use your new skills to solve. When learning is sequenced in the right manner, students can intentionally and systematically draw on their prior knowledge to address current challenges. For example, in figure 5.3, the first enduring understanding is "Health is affected by personal decisions and outside forces." The second is "Understanding pressures can help in making decisions." Being able to discuss the second enduring understanding is helped greatly by the first enduring understanding, because that understanding begins with the notion that individuals are decision makers and decisions are influenced by other people and forces. This makes the discussion of such pressures in the second enduring understanding considerably easier for the teacher to teach and for students to understand.

Learning progressions are valuable for teachers and students for these reasons:

- They identify must-know building blocks, enabling teachers to plan instructional sequences that give students systematic rather than sporadic opportunities to master each building block in the

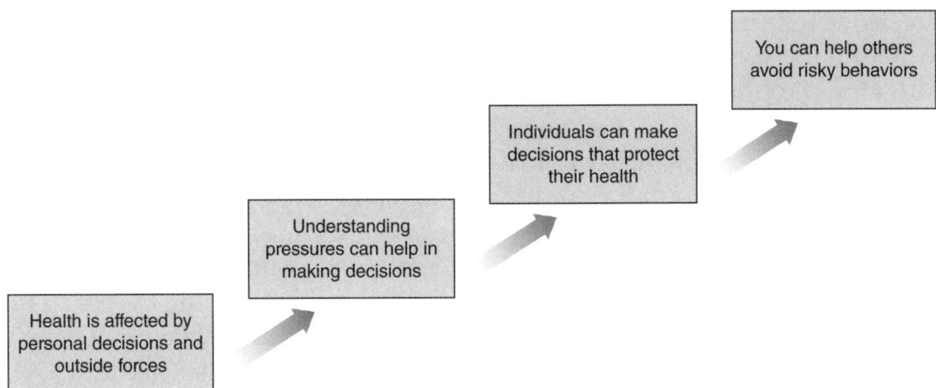

FIGURE 5.3   Four enduring understandings organized as learning progressions.

learning progression. If the teacher has a clear road map that designates pivotal stops along the way, it is far easier to incorporate those stops.

- Such analyses can form the framework for an optimal formative assessment process. Formative assessment provides evidence, routinely gathered during ongoing instruction, that helps teachers adjust their instruction and students adjust their learning tactics. Teachers can collect this adjustment-focused evidence using either formal or informal assessment techniques, but they should not collect such data on a whim. Rather, assessment should be thoughtfully planned.

- The formative assessment process will be far more successful if teachers systematically collect evidence of students' progress toward mastery of each key building block in a learning progression. If a student is having trouble with building blocks, assessments can pinpoint why. In the case of a student having trouble with a building block, assessment on the entire learning progression is unnecessary; it would be a waste of teacher–student time and would cause the teacher more planning time for reteaching in the future. We can look earlier in this chapter to Ms. Zeinz's example for proof of this.

How to Construct Learning Progressions

As was the case with the spiral curriculum, learning progressions are best constructed on the basis of a backward analysis. Teachers first identify a significant curricular outcome and ask, "What does a student need to know or be able to do to master this aim?" It is helpful to answer the question "What does a student need to know or be able to do?" in terms of building blocks of knowledge. Think about how you would teach someone to brush their teeth. You would start with the end of the process, washing the toothbrush with water. Then, you would work backwards, showing the physical motion of brushing teeth and where in the mouth to brush. Finally, you would teach how to put the toothpaste on the brush and run some water over the brush. In the example in figure 5.3, start at the last enduring understanding, the one at the top right, and look at how the three previous enduring understandings relate to each other.

Once the building blocks are identified, ask yourself, "What does a student need to know or be able to do to master this building block?" The answer to this question will lead to tasks and activities that can help teach the concepts, knowledge, and skills of a teaching block (see chapter 4).

Important Considerations in Designing Learning Progressions

The size of a building block is an important consideration. A general rule of thumb is that it is better to go smaller than larger to avoid overwhelming students with too much information at once. However, endless small building blocks, which may be unnecessary or could be combined, can interfere with both the pace of the lesson and student understanding.

Learning progressions should contain only those skills and knowledge that represent the most significant information needed to progress toward the enduring understanding. In figure 5.3, if you were to break the first enduring understanding ("Health is affected by personal decisions and outside forces") into building blocks, you might have four to six blocks consisting of concepts, knowledge, and skills such as (1) the concept of health status, or the sum of the positive and negative influences on a person's health and well-being; (2) the understanding that many factors influence your health status; (3) the principle that *health status* is affected by many factors, only some of which are controllable; and (4) the concept that decision-making affects your own health status. These building blocks of concepts, knowledge, and skills and the accompanying class activities (e.g., questioning activities, discussions, and debates; see chapter 4) allow the teacher and students to move incrementally toward the enduring understanding.

Selecting learning progressions and determining their size is a function of a teacher's experience. As a beginning teacher, consider the creation of learning progressions as similar to that of a sculptor who continues to shape his or her model, slightly refining each iteration. With each lesson you teach, you can make improvements. Given that you may teach the same lesson to many different classes throughout a day or over a term, this refinement can occur in a day, across a week, or from term to term. This is what it means to be adaptive and to learn from experience.

Summary

Both the spiral curriculum and learning progressions represent developmental, incremental, and recurrent dimensions of teaching. They are developmental in terms of meeting students where they are in their prior knowledge and developmental characteristics; incremental in terms of stepwise changes that occur sequentially and progressively; and recurrent in terms of revisiting the big idea, enduring understanding, or objectives across the curriculum. In the example of Ms. Zeinz, she decided to use both a spiral curriculum and learning progressions for her middle school health classes. Development of her spiral curriculum informed the development of her learning progressions. Today, she is less worried about student retention, and her teaching is more coherent and focused. She is now able to delve deeper into the content with each grade level.

CHAPTER 6

Teaching Health Content

Mr. Cortes is in his first two years of teaching. He wonders if he can arrange his lessons in ways that make use of what is known to be effective teaching. He starts the lesson by taking attendance, and then he discusses the purpose of the lesson. He teaches the content using questioning and experiential tasks, and he finishes with a closure. Though the types of tasks he asks students to do in each lesson are similar and he thinks they are good, he is unsatisfied with the structure of the lesson and feels that he is missing something.

What Mr. Cortes is reflecting on are ways of structuring lessons for repeated success. While this can be accomplished in many ways, none of which are the right way, the critical criterion is if the structure results in regular student learning. This can be true on some days and not on others. In this chapter we discuss components of the lesson that have been demonstrated by teaching practice and research to be overwhelmingly effective. Rosenshine (2012) found 10 teaching practices that have been shown to improve student learning consistently across all grade levels and most classroom subjects. (Physical education is an exception because it occurs outside the typical classroom setting.) Most of the practices have been discussed in other chapters (e.g., chapters 4 and 5), but in this chapter we focus on lessons rather than curriculum development. Rosenshine's (2012, p. 12) teaching practices are:

1. Begin the lesson with a short review of previous learning.
2. Present new material in small steps with student practice after each step.
3. Ask a large number of questions, and check the responses of all students.
4. Provide models that demonstrate thinking or procedures for solving problems.
5. Guide student practice as they begin to understand previously taught thinking and problem-solving strategies.
6. Check for understanding.
7. Obtain a high success rate in correct responses from your students.

8. Provide scaffolds for difficult tasks.
9. Require and monitor independent practice.
10. Engage students in weekly and monthly reviews.

Practice 1: Begin the Lesson With a Short Review of Previous Learning

Reviewing the previous work provides continuity with the current lesson and the unit. Reviewing previous work does not need to be a formal review by the teacher. It can occur in any of the following ways:

- Place question cards at each table in the classroom that ask students to discuss key elements of previous lessons as they enter the classroom.

- Help students recall the key elements of previous lessons by having a flash card quiz.

- A game show format (e.g., search the internet for the *Jeopardy* PowerPoint) is a fun way to review.

- Have students write their own questions at the end of the previous lesson to be used for this lesson. You then create a Kahoot with their questions. (Visit https://kahoot.com to set up a free account.)

- Ask students to create graphic organizers to link concepts and ideas together. (To see a variety of graphic organizers, visit https://creately.com/blog/diagrams/types-of-graphic-organizers/.)

- Ask students to share what they had difficulty with or to discuss where misunderstanding occurred or where errors were made with homework.

Practice 2: Present New Material in Small Steps With Student Practice After Each Step

In chapters 4 and 5 we talked about the importance of presenting content using small chunks of information incrementally and progressively. When content is grouped into small and easily digestible units of information, it is easier to comprehend. This approach of organizing content into small units is called chunking. Chunking is a teaching strategy used to reduce the cognitive load the learner is presented with in a lesson. Chunking occurs when you

- break large amounts of information into manageable information that is coherent,

- break projects or assignments into steps, and
- break a video longer than five minutes into several clips for discussion between segments.

Effective teachers spend time introducing the content to students in small chunks, taking time to provide multiple examples and models and to provide feedback. This approach takes up more lesson time because you are progressing more slowly as you cover the content in larger steps. However, this strategy is more effective at pulling along all the students and not just some. Each chunk should include accompanying activities for students to use or apply that knowledge or skill before moving to the next chunk. Observation of student use and application of knowledge and skills provides the teacher the opportunity to provide feedback and correct misunderstandings before the content progresses too far. In chapter 7 we examine this type of informal formative assessment.

A teacher who presents content using small chunks of information incrementally and progressively is like an archer slowly pulling back the string of a bow to shoot an arrow. The more carefully the teacher incrementally adds small chunks of information, the more likely students will be able to work independently. Their content comprehension will cover more ground, like an arrow.

Practice 3: Ask a Large Number of Questions, and Check the Responses of All Students

Questioning gives students practice at examining lesson content. Presenting their responses in their own words provides evidence that they are interacting with the content and not parroting back what they have heard. It also gives teachers an opportunity to discriminate and refine student answers. As such, questioning is a critical skill of effective teachers.

However, questioning can be conducted poorly and can result in poor student learning. For example, how often have you as a teacher or a student observed just one student responding to a question? This leads the teacher to wonder if other students in the class knew the answer. In many classrooms students who do not know the answer know that if they wait long enough someone who does know will speak up. The following are strategies that are designed to bypass the one-person answer outcome. Ask the question and have students write down their answers, and then

- hold up their answers on a card,
- share their answers with their table or group,
- discuss their answers with their table or group,
- have a competition among tables for the answer to the question, or
- read their answers in their journals collected weekly.

A second challenge of asking questions is whether one or two questions provide the teacher with enough of a sense that students understand. The solution here lies in understanding the types of questions you can ask. An instructor should ask questions that will require students to use the thinking skills the instructor is trying to develop. Bloom's Taxonomy is a hierarchical system for ordering thinking skills and creating specific questions to elicit lower- to higher-order thinking. For more information on Bloom's Taxonomy, we recommend the Illinois State University's education department website, listed in the references section.

In selecting questions, consider these guidelines:

- Focus on content that is considered essential knowledge.

- Use questions across the range of Bloom's Taxonomy with the specific intention of eliciting the level of responses you want to address.

- Ask questions that require an extended response. Avoid questions that can be answered with a simple yes or no unless you have planned follow-up questions.

- Script your questions and arrange them in a logical sequence (specific to general, lower level to higher level, a sequence related to content or skill steps).

- Your questions should not contain the answers. Avoid implied response questions when you are genuinely seeking an answer from the class. A question such as "Don't we all agree?" will not encourage student response.

An important aspect of classroom interaction is the manner in which the teacher handles student responses. When an instructor asks a question, (1) students can respond, which gives the teacher an opportunity to reinforce the answer, correct the answer, or probe for more information; (2) students can ask a question that provides an opportunity for teachers to clarify their question; or (3) students can give no response. In this situation, calling on students by name and pausing and waiting for an answer are good strategies.

Practice 4: Provide Models That Demonstrate Thinking or Procedures for Solving Problems

Providing students with models, examples, or demonstrations helps them to generalize problem-solving. By this we mean that students can copy the model and apply it to novel situations. Imagine learning to drive without ever having seen a person drive. It would take longer to understand how to solve the problems of driving. Models make procedures and thinking visible by allowing students to observe the teacher's thought processes as they resolve problems. Using this type of instruction, teachers engage students in the imitation of particular behaviors, which students can then apply to other situations and problems, particularly when they are working on their own independent practice or homework.

Consider the following when modeling:

- Be sure to connect to prior knowledge.
- Use chunking, and teach in an incremental and progressive manner.
- Provide visual, auditory, kinesthetic, and tactile ways to illustrate the concept, knowledge, or skill.
- Think aloud as you demonstrate each step.
- In your description, be sure to emphasize the connections throughout each step.
- Check repeatedly for understanding.
- Provide more than one example in your modeling.
- Allow students opportunities to ask questions and get clarification.

Practice 5: Guide Student Practice as They Begin to Understand Previously Taught Thinking and Problem-Solving Strategies

Guided practice is an instructional strategy that moves students from observing the teacher modeling the task, to performing the task under close supervision so feedback can occur and questions can be answered, to being able to perform the task in independent practice. In short, it is the link between modeling and independent practice. A number of arguments have been made that this link is unnecessary and that students should learn on their own. However, as Clark, Kirschner, and Sweller (2012, p. 6) note, "Decades of research clearly demonstrate that for novices (comprising virtually all students), direct, explicit instruction is more effective and more efficient than partial guidance." Importantly, Rosenshine (2012, p. 17), in his review of the research on guided practice, observed, "The most successful teachers spent more time in guided practice, more time asking questions, more time checking for understanding, and more time correcting errors."

The goal of guided practice is for the role of the teacher to shift from direct instruction of the content (modeling), where students are reliant on the teacher for learning, to facilitating, assisting, and supporting students in guided practice as they begin the work with guidance, to monitoring students as they work in independent practice.

Here are six ways to guide students:

1. Create time when students can ask questions to clarify the task.
2. Encourage students to return to the guidelines of the task. This will require that you have guidelines they can see on a PowerPoint slide, paper, or other visual platform.
3. Ask students to think aloud by describing to a peer, small group, or the class what they are doing.
4. Ask lots of questions of students.
5. Discuss correct and incorrect responses with students and, in particular, the "why" of their incorrect responses.
6. Promote reflecting on learning. Have regular times in the lesson when students reflect on what they have learned.

Table 6.1 presents the roles of the students and teacher during guided practice.

TABLE 6.1   Roles for Students and Teachers During Guided Practice

Students	Teachers
Imitate models that have been taught, and use them to solve similar and then different problems.	Clearly describe the task to students.
Participate in questioning, discussion, and problem-solving with peers in small groups or with partners or teachers.	Create discussion and work activities that encourage questioning, and focus students on the critical steps described in the model.
Receive and use feedback.	Monitor students' understanding of skills and concepts.

Practice 6: Check for Understanding

In many of the teaching practices in this chapter (e.g., guided practice and modeling) checking for understanding is a key element. Checking for understanding requires that the teacher regularly check in with students during the lesson to verify that they understand what is being taught. Many ways to check for understanding, such as the questioning strategies, have been discussed earlier in this chapter. Here are some more ways to check for understanding:

- Students write a summary of the main idea in one or two sentences and share this with a neighbor.

- Students raise their hands if they agree with the answer that someone else has given.
- Students rate their understanding on a scale from 1 to 10.
- Ask students to explain the concept to a partner.
- Ask students to compare and contrast concepts with a partner.
- Ask students to create a concept map (see teach.its.uiowa.edu).
- Ask students what frustrates and confuses them about the content and why.
- Ask students to create an outline; you will first have to teach them what an outline is.
- Give a short (few questions) quiz.
- Have students quiz the teacher.
- Ask students to fill in worksheets with key descriptors or terms left blank (e.g., guided notes).

Practice 7: Obtain a High Success Rate in Correct Responses From Your Students

This may sound obvious, but it is important that students are successful in class. The single most important factor in predicting whether a student will learn and be successful in school is if they understand the content they have been taught. One criterion to determine this is their answers to questions posed by the teacher. Teachers who quickly respond to errors are more effective. A high percentage of successful answers conversely indicates a low error rate. Research has revealed that classes with the teachers most successful at producing student learning typically have students respond with more than 80 percent correct answers (Rosenshine 2012).

Recognizing and responding to student errors appropriately is one of the main tasks of teachers. Teachers should correct student misunderstanding and errors. However, errors should not be seen as dead ends but rather as potential avenues to explore student misunderstanding of the content. Teachers should move beyond right or wrong answers given by students and instead should use student misunderstanding as opportunities to help students improve their understanding of the conceptual basis of their errors and to improve their critical thinking (Ball 1990).

Obtaining high success rates from your students is among the most important educational outcomes for a teacher. Using the teaching practices described in this chapter is a strong first step toward achieving this.

Practice 8: Provide Scaffolds for Difficult Tasks

In construction, a scaffold is a temporary structure used to support a work crew on a building project (e.g., planks that allow painters to paint the outside of a tall building). In education, scaffolding is an approach that provides the learner support as they move from learning to independent practice. Using scaffolds in this way is a form of guided practice and should be used specifically for difficult tasks. Examples of scaffolds that can support students include the following:

- Break a task into smaller parts. Refer to chunking, discussed earlier in the chapter.
- Use think-aloud strategies for both teacher and students. For example, ask students to complete sentences or answer questions such as
  - What have you learned so far?
  - What didn't make sense?
  - What do you think will happen next?
  - I was confused by . . .
  - What is the most important part of . . .
  - What was interesting in this?
- Use visual aids such as graphic organizers, videos, pictures, and charts to provide visual models of the health content.
- Use discussion strategies. (See chapter 10 for details.)
- Use active learning strategies such as asking students to write down the important facts, findings, or key points from what they are reading, talking about, or watching.

Practice 9: Require and Monitor Independent Practice

As described previously, independent practice follows guided practice in a lesson. It occurs when the teacher asks students to work on their own with little to no assistance. Independent practice's primary purpose is to allow students many opportunities to apply the knowledge and skills taught by the teacher and developed in guided practice to be honed so that guidance is no longer needed.

Independent practice is grounded in the idea that students need a lot of deliberate practice. You would not expect a student to perform a layup once and then be able to perform it well every time after that. Similarly, learning and applying health education knowledge and skills requires a lot of intentional and systematic practice with varied health examples. This results in overlearning and is evidenced by students who can perform the tasks fluently. When this happens students can then devote more of their attention to using their newly acquired knowledge and skills in more challenging tasks or building blocks.

Some important considerations for the use of independent practice include the following:

- Before moving to independent practice, teachers must be assured that students understand and have the competence to apply the health knowledge and skills they have learned. This requires some formative assessment in guided practice to provide evidence that students are ready to move to independent practice. Chapter 7 discusses formative assessment strategies that can be used for this purpose.

- The tasks that students are asked to do in independent practice should be systematically varied in terms of increasing difficulty and differing situations. Teachers should use several tasks rather than just one or two and assuming that students can do all relevant tasks.

- Homework is an example of independent practice and should be a key part of every lesson, because developing students' competence and independence requires time and effort.

- The tasks that students can do in independent practice include assignments, projects, and the like.

- Independent practice does not mean that the teacher leaves students alone. It does not involve ignoring students as they work. Independent practice should be monitored, and the teacher should step in to assist students when they ask for help or are struggling.

Practice 10: Engage Students in Weekly and Monthly Reviews

A critical element of teaching lies in making sense of the content and connecting past content to that currently being taught. In chapter 5 we discussed the benefits of the spiral curriculum and its design, which allows teachers and students to revisit prior learning to leverage it for current learning. The more students revisit content and make connections with what they are learning today, the stronger these interconnections become. One way to do this beyond the spiral curriculum is to use weekly and monthly reviews.

Content can be reviewed using the following strategies:

- Make connections by using the same cues, prompts, and language in your reviews.
- Use regular short tests and other forms of assessment.
- Have students write an outline, notes, or a graphic organizer. Graphic organizers can help show relationships of concepts and the scope of the work. Graphic organizers can be used in two ways. The first is to ask students to write one from scratch to show how they understand the relationships. The second is to incorporate a graphic organizer showing only the past content that has been previously covered and what is currently being taught. Then ask students to reproduce the graphic organizer each week or month and have them explain to their partner or group what the concepts mean.
- Students can teach their peers to provide evidence of what they have learned.

Summary

Today, Mr. Cortes doesn't use all of this chapter's teaching practices in each lesson he teaches. He does use most of them daily, though, and they are all present each week in his lessons. Mr. Cortes has confidence in using these practices, because they work and are undergirded by strong research base. However, when he first started using the practices, he experienced a small learning curve to be able to use them effectively. Give yourself time to learn how best to make these practices work in your lessons, day by day and week by week, with the knowledge that these practices will result in stronger lessons.

CHAPTER 7

Assessing Learning

Ms. Kim's seventh-grade health class is at the midway point of a series of lessons focused on human physiology. The goal of the current lesson is for students to understand the energy systems and to access valid information about them. Prior to this lesson, students had finished a unit on nutrition and goal setting. In her review of the nutrition content to start the next unit, her discussion led her to realize that many of the students demonstrated some misconceptions about macronutrients (e.g., protein, carbohydrate, and fat). Ms. Kim is frustrated by this misunderstanding. She is going to have to revisit the nutrition content before moving forward with the energy systems unit, and this will put her behind schedule. In conversation with her mentor, Mr. Morgan, the issue of how she knew that her students had learned the content of the lessons was a large part of their discussion. Upon reflection, Ms. Kim indicated that she did not do any unit assessments and that she was waiting to assess all content at the end of the term. As she said this, she realized she was not using assessment correctly.

Assessment is a central part of instruction. Student assessment is essential to (1) measure the progress and performance of individual students by comparing their learning against outcomes and standards; (2) gather evidence about students' knowledge, understanding, and skills to inform the planning of future instruction; and (3) share information with relevant stakeholders. Assessment can be categorized broadly in two ways: summative and formative assessment.

Summative Assessment

Summative assessments include tests, quizzes, and other course activities such as projects and assignments that are used to measure the cumulative understanding students have acquired over a unit or at the end of a course of study. To use a gardening analogy, summative assessment is similar to a gardener collecting flowers after a season of growth. The collection of flowers does not affect the growth of the flowers; one is simply collecting the flowers. At the end of the collection, the gardener might say, "These flowers are much bigger (or smaller) than last year" or "These flowers have lost their fragrance." But the collection of the flowers does not affect the size or fragrance. Similarly, with summative assessments, teachers collect data to determine where a student is, not how or why the student got to where he or she is. They are not collecting data about the journey. They could compare the data to previously collected data, but that does not tell them what made for any differences or similarities. Therefore, summative assessments are defined by three criteria:

1. The assessments (e.g., tests, assignments, or projects) are used to determine whether students have learned what they were expected to learn. In other words, what makes an assessment summative is not the design of the assessment, but its purpose, which is to determine to what degree students have learned the content they have been taught.

2. They are evaluative rather than diagnostic. They are more appropriately used to determine learning progress and achievement, evaluate the effectiveness of educational programs, measure progress toward improvement goals, or to make course-placement decisions.

3. Their results are typically used to determine grades.

Unlike summative assessments in reading or mathematics, very few standardized tests are available for health educators. This means that, for the most part, the tests used by teachers for summative purposes are teacher made. Table 7.1 discusses the major forms of summative assessments as well as their advantages and disadvantages.

TABLE 7.1   Types of Summative Evaluations

	Description	Advantages	Disadvantages
Multiple-choice tests	Students choose one or more items from a limited list of choices. A multiple-choice question consists of a stem, the correct answer, and typically three to four incorrect or less correct answers.	• You can ask more questions than in short answer tests and therefore assess more content. • It takes less time to complete a multiple-choice question compared to a short answer test. • They are the easiest to grade. • Students do not have to formulate an answer but can focus on discriminating the correct answer from among the choices.	• They offer limited feedback to correct errors in student understanding. • They tend to focus on low-level learning objectives. • Development of good test items is time consuming. • Measuring the ability to organize and express ideas is not possible.

Table 7.1   *(continued)*

	Description	**Advantages**	**Disadvantages**
Peer assessment	A pair or group of students assess each other's work using a rubric or criteria previously determined by the teacher or students.	• It encourages student responsibility and ownership. • Students develop skills of judgment. • It offers a valuable alternative feedback perspective, especially for teamwork and behavior.	• Grade inflation is likely. • Students may be reluctant to give negative feedback if not anonymous. • Teachers are required to train students on how to assess and give feedback. • Teacher supervision may take teacher time or attention away from other important things.
Self-assessment	Students make judgments about their own learning, achievements, and learning outcomes, usually according to established criteria.	• Students develop skills of judgment. • It encourages goal setting and responsibility. • It promotes the development of reflective practice.	• Grade inflation is likely. • Guided practice is required to develop self-monitoring skills.

Formative Assessment

The Council of Chief State School Officers (2018, p. 2) defines formative assessment as "a planned, ongoing process used by all students and teachers during learning and teaching to elicit and use evidence of student learning to improve student understanding of intended disciplinary learning outcomes and support students to become self-directed learners." Formative assessment is used to measure student learning continuously throughout a unit of instruction. Using the gardening analogy from the beginning of the chapter, formative assessment is like feeding and watering plants as needed to ensure they continue to grow. Formative assessment has a variety of strategies that can be used to evaluate the effects of your instruction on a daily and ongoing basis. Formative assessments reveal how and what students are learning during the lesson or unit and can be used to inform the next steps in instruction.

Effective use of the formative assessment process requires students and teachers to integrate and embed the following practices into a collaborative and respectful classroom environment:

- Clarifying learning goals and success criteria within a broader progression of learning
- Eliciting and analyzing evidence of student thinking

- Engaging in self-assessment and peer feedback
- Providing actionable feedback
- Using evidence and feedback to move learning forward by adjusting learning strategies, goals, or next instructional steps (The Council of Chief State School Officers 2018, p. 2).

The following ideas are a few techniques for providing formative assessments to your students.

Entry and Exit Slips

The entry and exit slip strategy helps students summarize and reflect on information learned in a class. Exit slips give students an opportunity to review keys ideas, consider essential details, and summarize their thinking. Students respond to one to three teacher questions that focus on the content of the lesson. Exit slip questions can also focus on the process of learning or on the effectiveness of a teaching methodology. Responses to these questions give an informal measure of each student's understanding of the lesson or concept, allowing the teacher to plan for the next lesson. Similarly, entry slips can be used to connect content learned in the last lesson or prior knowledge as a review. Entry and exit slips should be used as a routine, and they work best when the questions are specific (e.g., "What is the take home message from our glitter example in today's communicable diseases lesson?") rather than general statements (e.g., "What did you learn today?"). A good source for entry and exit slip templates is theteachertoolkit.com. A quick way to see the big picture if you use paper entry and exit slips is to sort the papers into three piles: those who got the point, those who sort of got it, and those who didn't get it. The size of the stacks is your clue about what to do next. Filtering through student answers will also help you shape your future instruction, especially for those students who are not grasping the content easily.

Technology

Using online technology for polls and quizzes can help you get a better sense of how much they really understand. These can be created with apps like Socrative, Nearpod, or Quizlet, or with in-class games and tools such as Quizalize, Kahoot, FlipQuiz, Gimkit, Plickers, or Flippity. Among these tools' advantages is that they are an efficient way to monitor and evaluate learning while delivering fun and engaging interactions for learners. Because you can design the questions yourself, you determine the level of difficulty and complexity. Importantly, they record the responses of all of your students, allowing you an easy way to determine prior knowledge and to track progress both individually and in aggregate. You can assign low point values to these quizzes for motivation. If these are used on a weekly or daily routine, they become an excellent tool for teachers and a motivation for students.

Dipsticks

Dipsticks, derived from the quick and easy way of checking the oil in your car, are time-efficient ways to check for understanding. Entry and exit slips are one example of a dipstick. Here are some others:

- Ask students to draw what they just learned, to visually represent their understanding.
- Have students write down an explanation of what they understand.
- Ask students to write two or three questions they have about the topic.
- Ask students to give a thumbs-up, middle thumb, or thumbs-down to rate their understanding.
- Have students raise their hands if they agree with the answer that someone else has given.
- Ask students to rate their understanding on a scale from 1 to 10.
- Ask students to compare and contrast concepts with a partner.
- Ask students what frustrates and confuses them about the content and why.
- Ask students to create an outline; you will first have to teach them what an outline is.
- Give a short (few questions) quiz.
- Have students quiz the teacher.
- Ask students to fill in worksheets with key descriptors or terms left blank (e.g., guided notes).

These can be collected and easily judged using the three-pile sorting method described earlier.

Misconceptions and Errors

Sometimes it is helpful to see if students understand why something is incorrect or why a concept is hard. Ask students to explain the most confusing or the hardest part of the lesson. Alternatively, present students with a common misunderstanding or error and ask them to correct the misunderstanding or error.

Open-Ended Questions

These questions get students writing or talking about the topic for a range or fixed period of time (e.g., 3-10 minutes or 10 minutes). Avoid yes-or-no questions and phrases like "Does this make sense?" Open-ended questions require students to answer in complete sentences.

Quizzes

Give a short quiz at the end of class. Some great ways to give quizzes can be found at www.leadquizzes.com or www.teachthought.com.

Summary of the Main Idea

Ask students to write a summary of the main idea in one or two sentences and share this with a neighbor. You could also have students summarize or paraphrase important concepts and lessons orally, visually, or using technology.

Think-Pair-Share

This strategy is a collaborative learning activity during which students work together to solve a problem or answer a question. This strategy requires students to think individually about a topic or answer to a question and to share ideas with classmates. Discussing with a partner maximizes participation, focuses attention, and engages students in comprehending the reading material. The procedure for this activity follows:

Think

You begin by asking a specific question. Students are given a specific amount of time to think about what their response is. They can also make notes as they think.

Pair

Each student should have been previously paired with another student or a small group (e.g., a table).

Share

Students share their thinking with their partner or group. You can expand the sharing time into a whole-class discussion.

One-Question Quiz

You ask a single focused question, with a specific goal response, that can be answered within a minute or two. You can quickly scan the written responses to assess student understanding.

Concept Maps

These are a graphic representation of students' knowledge and provide you with insights into how students organize and represent knowledge. (See https://teach.its.uiowa.edu for more on concept maps.)

Concept maps are a useful strategy for assessing both the knowledge students have coming into a program or course and their developing knowledge of course material. Concept maps include concepts, usually enclosed in circles or boxes, and relationships between concepts, indicated by a connecting line. Words on the line are linking words and specify the relationship between concepts. These can also be created using the Popplet website or app.

Considerations in the Use of Summative and Formative Assessment

As you develop methods for assessing your students, consider the following:

- Teachers should use both formative and summative assessments. It is important to know what is happening during instruction and at the end of the lesson or unit.

- Be sure that the assessment is developed before you develop the instruction, so the instruction is aligned with the assessment. Too often assessments are designed after the instruction is developed, resulting in disconnections that confuse students, which then prevents the teacher from gathering valuable information on their next steps. Assessment outcomes and goals should drive the instruction that is to occur.

- Make sure that your use of formative assessment is sustainable over time and that you actually use the assessment to inform instruction.

- Use the results of summative assessments to improve the unit of instruction. You will more than likely teach a unit over and over in your career. Each time you teach it, you should be updating and improving the unit. You can add physical or electronic sticky notes to your existing assessments for revision in the future, or you can make the changes right away for next time.

Summary

For many teachers, assessment may appear onerous and time-consuming. It certainly can be, but it doesn't have to be. Formative assessment allows teachers to adapt their instruction as a result of what students are learning. The strategies described in this chapter represent some of the many ways teachers can determine what students know and are able to do and thus how effective their instruction is. They can be used frequently and routinely in each lesson and can be evaluated by the teacher efficiently and easily. Formative assessment should drive the instruction in the lesson because it provides immediate feedback on student understanding. Every year more and more technology is available to help teachers with formative assessment. Among the advantages of technology is that a record of individual and class performance is kept and is immediately available to the teacher. Summative assessment is used to determine understanding at the end of a unit of instruction and is often used to assign grades, but it should also be used to redesign units of instruction if trends are revealed in student understanding or misunderstanding in the summative assessment. When Ms. Kim evaluated the lack of use of formative and summative assessments, she realized that not only is it an aid to her as a teacher but that it is not particularly challenging to create or to incorporate into her lessons.

Pedagogical Considerations

Creating Expectations Using Rules and Managerial Routines

It is a Saturday morning, and Mr. Barnham is stressed as he reflects on the state of his teaching of health education. He is frustrated that his lessons are interrupted by recurring events he feels should not be occurring in his class. He has rules for the students to follow, but it seems that he needs many more rules in order to deal with what is going on in his classroom. Issues such as students needing to sharpen their pencils, getting tissues to blow their nose, deciding where to sit in each lesson, getting up and moving to the door when the bell rings before he actually dismisses them are disruptions that occur on a daily basis. He is also dealing with students who are not motivated to be in health class. Collectively, these individual events disrupt his delivery of the lesson. He is tired of revisiting the same challenges each day, and he is fearful of accepting them for the rest of his career.

Mr. Barnham is not alone in feeling frustrated about classroom management. Managerial challenges are reported as the second most important issue of concern for teachers (Ingersoll and Smith 2004). Consider for a moment the message you might internalize as a health teacher if each day you encounter the same challenges and each day they frustrate you. Not all challenges can be removed. For example, students with particular individualized education plans (IEPs) may present recurring challenges as you work to accommodate them. In this chapter we discuss how to remove or minimize most challenges that interrupt the flow of the health lesson so that you can be less stressed and that students can learn more effectively and efficiently. The chapter is organized around three beliefs:

1. Your classroom is a culture. It should be fair and kind, but it should be businesslike in that it is clear why everyone is there—to learn health education.

2. Students should rehearse the rules and routines to learn the culture, and periodically you will need to revisit these rules and routines to reteach or refine them over time.

3. Rules and procedures are critical managerial components, but you need a system that brings it all together and engages students to ensure lessons move forward.

The Class Climate You Want for Teaching Health Education

When we talk to teachers, they often tell us they did not get into teaching to spend a lot of their time on classroom management activities, and they often wonder if they need to be doing management all the time. Yet, quality classroom environments seldom exhibit many disciplinary actions by the teacher. Instead, in an organized classroom, students are on task and know what to do. But this does not mean that the teacher did not specifically create that environment. Walter Doyle (1986), an educational researcher, argued that teachers need to acquire and keep control of their classes and that getting the cooperation of the students is central to this. Figure 8.1 shows three points along a continuum of classroom culture. At one end of the continuum, students are noncompliant, which includes behaviors such as not listening, talking when the teacher is talking, being off task, moving on tasks too slowly, and not contributing to the class.

The middle point on the continuum, compliant, means that students follow directions, are on task, complete their work individually and in groups, and are respectful of each other and the teacher.

The third point is the cooperative classroom. Students are not only compliant, but they actively contribute to the classroom culture by making suggestions, being proactive such as cleaning up after themselves without being prompted, and exceeding the expectations of the teacher. They own the lessons with the teacher. This third stage is also characterized by increased student decision-making, which in turn leads to increased student engagement in the lesson.

In this chapter, everything we discuss is focused on helping you create a cooperative culture in your classroom, which, of course, is what all

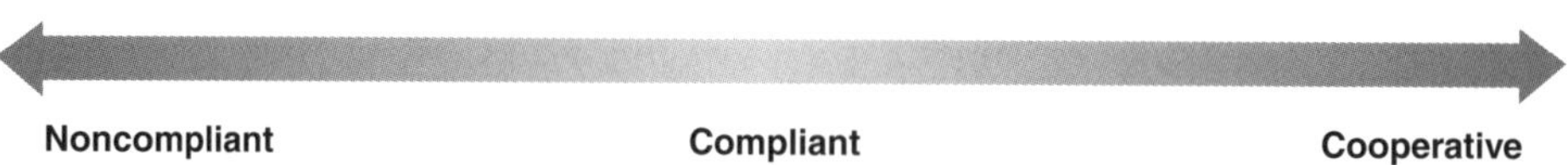

FIGURE 8.1 The continuum of classroom culture.

teachers want for their classroom. This is achieved by creating expectations of your culture that are initially formed by your rules and managerial routines.

Rules in a Health Education Classroom

Rules define the basic conduct of students in your classroom. Some general principles should be considered regarding rules (Alter and Haydon 2017), and they work best when

- there are few of them, ideally between four and seven;
- they are specific and clear in what is meant by the rule;
- they are posted in the classroom for all to see;
- they are tied to positive and negative consequences; and
- students are engaged in formulating them.

Tables 8.1 and 8.2 provide examples of rules for elementary and secondary classrooms. Each rule presents a similar set of tasks, but the way they are written varies. There is no right way; it is simply a matter of your style and the type of culture you want to present.

TABLE 8.1   Examples of Rules for Elementary Classrooms

Example A	Example B	Example C
Show respect.	Be kind; say please and thank you.	Take care of yourself by being prepared for work and paying attention to the teacher and your classmates.
Put forth your best effort.	Listen to the teacher and classmates.	Take care of others by sharing, listening to them, helping them, and keeping your hands to yourself.
Be prepared to learn.	Follow directions.	Take care of the environment by leaving things better than how you found them when you clean up or organize.
Be positive.	Do your best.	Have an attitude that leads to success; turn your work in on time.
Pay attention and ask questions.	Take risks and make mistakes.	Be creative.
Take responsibility for your actions.	Make good choices.	—

TABLE 8.2 Examples of Rules for Secondary Classrooms

Example A	Example B	Example C
Come to class prepared to learn, with sharpened pencils, pen, paper, and notebooks.	Be on time and on task.	Be punctual; arrive on time to class.
Respect all property (school, personal, and others' property).	Take responsibility and be proactive.	Be polite to everyone.
Respect all discussions in class and do not criticize anybody's ideas or opinions.	Respect your teacher, your classmates, and the classroom.	Be prompt with your homework each day.
Do your very best!	Be here; all technology needs to be put away unless we are using it.	Be prepared to work.
—	—	Be productive.

Positive and Negative Consequences With Rules

A number of principles should be followed when using positive and negative consequences. It is important to focus mostly on positive consequences. Here are some important tasks for teachers:

- Rehearse examples of the rules. Provide students with examples, and have them practice following the rules.
- Allow students to self-correct and redo if they ignore a rule. You can help by prompting and creating opportunities for redos.
- Praise accomplishment of the rules regularly, but initially do so a lot. If a student is not following a rule, praise the students who are complying rather than focusing on the student who is not.
- By all means praise, but if praise alone is not working, use bigger reinforcers such as free time or award points that give access to things students would like to do.
- Set a goal for students as the class starts or establish a contract with students to follow the rules.

Negative consequences should be used only when the above positives do not work well, but the teacher should still focus on being positive when the rules are followed. The best consequences are reasonable and logical, and should move along a continuum from light to stronger consequences. A teacher might follow this sequence:

- Ask the student to perform the rule-following behavior when they do not.

- Have the student be the last to leave the class.
- Deprive the student of some reward.
- Issue the student a time-out.
- Send the student to detention.

Routines

Effective classroom teaching requires organization of the physical environment. The physical environment affects motivation and the pace of learning in lessons, and includes such considerations as desk and table orientation, the establishment of work areas, the attractiveness of the classroom, and the arrangement of media. Classroom routines and procedures are taught to students and recur in the classroom every day. They include the following.

Routines for Arrival and Dismissal

Routines for arrival and dismissal reduce delays in the start of class, free the teacher to deal with interactions that require special attention, ensure that classes end smoothly, allow students to leave on time, and give the teacher time to set the classroom up for the next class.

Routines for Handling Transitions and Interruptions

Events such as arriving late to class with or without a pass or returning to the room from the nurse or restroom can disrupt an already running class and can break everyone's focus. A classroom will always have individuals who for one reason or another are late to class. Do not fight it; rather, establish a routine.

Routines for Dealing With Materials and Equipment

Having routines for distributing and collecting materials and homework, sharpening pencils, and getting a tissue ensure that the class will not have to be interrupted. Additionally, these routines entrust students with resolving the problem.

Routines for Managing Group Work

How to form teams, moving to work areas, expected behaviors as a member of the group, communication strategies within and between groups and with the teacher are all routines that occur in groups. More time is lost each day putting students into groups than many other managerial issues. Having a routine to do this will save a lot of time, keep the lesson moving forward, and again allow students to know that you trust they can follow the routine.

Routines for Seatwork and Teacher-Led Activities

It is helpful to establish routines for how students take notes, participate in classwork, help peers or ask for help, and what students should do when work is completed. For example, for how to behave when listening to the teacher during instruction, we recommend using the acronym SLANT:

Sit up

Listen

Ask and answer questions

Take **n**otes

Track the speaker

This routine is gold. It helps students organize their understanding of the lesson.

Six Strategies for Teaching Routines

Students do not enter your class knowing your routines. In fact, each of their classrooms likely follows a different routine. Routines need to be taught and should be revisited periodically. Here are six strategies to teach routines:

1. Explain why you want the routine. For example, "We are doing this so that I do not have to tell you what to do each day and so that you can have more responsibility in the class."
2. Model what you want to see.
3. Specify what you do not want to see.
4. Rehearse on the first few days what you want.
5. Use whatever accountability method you wish, but we recommend using points. Award bonus points for completing the routines over the first few weeks of school, and periodically award points across the year to teams that are following routines well.
6. Practice the routine periodically or when performance slips.

Using a System to Organize Your Health Education Classroom

In order to manage all of the class routines and to facilitate a cooperative classroom in which the students are engaged in the success of the lesson, it is helpful to use a system. One system we recommend is borrowed from

Example of a Managerial System

Students enter the classroom, return their homework to the homework basket (one basket per class), and then move to their assigned seats with their teams of four or five peers. Each team has its own table and affiliation. In this health unit, the students have chosen their own team names (e.g., Scallywags, Nutritionists, Pirates, Giraffes).

As students return to their seats, one student at each table, designated as the organizer, walks to the teacher's table and retrieves a folder of work for their team. When the organizer returns to the team table, he or she hands each team member an entry slip with questions about what was learned in the last lesson or sometimes a survey seeking student input on things like how they are perceiving or valuing the lesson content or suggestions of topics to focus on next. Students complete the entry slip.

Simultaneously, a team member called the recordkeeper takes attendance using an attendance sheet with the names of the group on it and hands it to the teacher once everyone in the group has arrived. The teacher can double-check this with a glance when submitting their attendance report to the school. During this time, the teacher does not direct the work of the students. The students follow a series of routines, and the teacher is free to meet with individual students as needed or move from group to group to check on progress.

Once the introductory routines of the lesson are complete, the teacher may choose to start the lesson with a lecture or give the captains (or cocaptain if the captain is not present) of each team a task for their team to do. The teacher describes the task to the whole class, and the captains are responsible for ensuring their team is on task, or the teacher may call the captains over while the entry task is being completed and describe the task to the captains, who then return to their teams and describe the task to their teammates.

After the task is completed, the teacher asks questions of the class. Each captain then leads a discussion with their group based on the teacher's instructions. When the team is required to share with the class, the organizer reports the team's findings. In the course of the lesson, teams receive points for being on task, following rules and routines, completing work, performing their roles, cooperating, and contributing to the lesson.

The recordkeeper keeps track of these points and at the end of class adds them to the team chart. These points are used for motivation and can be used to assess student performance. The points accumulate throughout the unit of instruction in health education, and at the end of the unit or a series of units, the teams can win awards such as free time, reading time, prizes from a mystery bag, and visitors. At times during the lesson the teacher may give individual and group quizzes, and it is the recordkeeper in each group who hands out the tests and collects them.

A lesson can take several forms including group projects, direct instruction, peer learning, and cooperative learning, but whatever the form, the team typically works together or is broken into smaller subgroups as needed. As the lesson comes to a close the organizer gives each student in the team an exit slip with specific questions about the lesson.

a physical education curriculum model called sport education (Siedentop, Hastie, and van der Mars 2020). This model works well in elementary through secondary classes and is organizational, motivational, and instructional. As you read the Example of a Managerial System sidebar, look for the many procedures already mentioned in this chapter.

You should be able to see many of the routines discussed in this chapter occurring in the model. The model works for several reasons, but key among these are that the students are involved in making the lesson work, they have responsibilities as team leaders, and there is little teacher involvement in beginning the lesson because of the routines. Entry slips provide connection to previous work, and most importantly, the pace of the lesson does not require wait time. If you use this system you will need to do the following tasks.

Assign Students to Teams of Four or Five

In selecting the students, distribute them as equally as you can relative to ability, gender, and behavioral characteristics so that it is as close to a level playing field for each team as possible. The students will stay in the same groups for the duration of their time with you (weeks, semester, or year). You reserve the right to make changes to maintain equity across teams, but such changes should occur early in the first unit.

Assign Names to Teams

Teachers can either assign team names such as the ones listed in table 8.3 or have students create their own team names such as the ones at the beginning of the sidebar.

TABLE 8.3   Sample Team Names

Example A	Example B
Energizers	Centers for Disease Control
Retrofitters	American Medical Association
Esprit	American Public Health Association
Positive Pulse	National Institute of Mental Health
Vitality	World Health Organization
Wellness	American Medical Association

	Description	Advantages	Disadvantages
Short answer tests	Students answer structured questions with an open-ended response. They are scored against predetermined model answers.	• They are easy to create. • They are easier to grade than full essays. • The answer is not in front of the student, who must construct a response instead of selecting a response from multiple choices.	• Because short answers require time, less content is assessed compared to multiple-choice exams.
Essay and report	Students submit prose in response to a set of questions or a topic. They can be scored either with a points system against a rubric or using a global rating.	• They are easy to create. • They can assess written communication skills. • They allow the assessment of complex topics and ability to make coherent arguments. • They can demonstrate understanding of the interrelationships of concepts.	• They offer limited coverage of content. • They are time-consuming to grade.
Oral questioning, presentations, and performance	Teacher or peers ask questions of a student. The student makes a presentation on a topic or performs an experiment or demonstration of a concept. These can be graded using a predetermined rubric.	• Students can show or demonstrate what they know. • They are adaptable to student need.	• They offer limited assessment of content. • They are time-consuming to conduct. • They can be stressful for students. • They can be hard to grade.
Portfolio or projects	A portfolio is a collection of work samples, projects, and evaluations.	• Portfolios and projects allow for the assessment of complex tasks and for different types of student work. • They encourage student reflection on learning. Students may come to understand what they have and have not learned. • They are adaptable to student need.	• They are time-consuming for students to create and for teachers to grade. • They can be more difficult to grade. • They often are poorly accepted by students. • Class time is required to prepare the portfolio assignment or project and to assist students. • Students must retain and compile their own work, usually outside of class. Motivating students to create the portfolio may be difficult. • Students who recently transferred to the class may have difficulty meeting portfolio requirements.

(continued)

Create Roles With Leadership Responsibilities

In the previous sidebar we discussed the roles of captain, organizer, recordkeeper, and cocaptain. Here are the specific responsibilities for each role:

The *captain/cocaptain* is responsible for

- working with other teams when instruction requires teams to interact (e.g., debates, jigsaw puzzles, and competitions),
- keeping the group on task with encouragement,
- motivating the team with prompts,
- meeting with the teacher for tasks, and
- describing tasks to and sharing the goals of the tasks with their team.

The *organizer* is responsible for

- handing out entry and exit slips,
- collecting materials for the lesson,
- organizing cleanup at the end of the lesson, and
- making sure materials are returned by team members.

The *recordkeeper* is responsible for

- tracking group tasks,
- recording assessment points,
- managing quizzes and handing them in to the teacher,
- taking attendance, and
- website updates.

The *cocaptain* is responsible for

- taking on the role of anyone who is not present,
- acting as captain of one of the subgroups if the group splits, and
- helping any group member with tasks.

You can use whatever titles you like for different tasks, and you may want to add additional roles, especially if teams have more than four members. The essential feature of this system is that students stay in the same teams for the duration of their time with you. You can rotate the roles among the team members for each unit, but we recommend not doing this within a unit. Students are given responsibilities for helping the lesson progress, which gives them some ownership of the lesson and in doing so creates positive peer support. The system creates a cooperative work environment that frees the teacher to teach the lesson.

Create Accountability

For accountability we recommend using a PowerPoint or Word file to create a chart like the one in figure 8.2, one for each team. This chart can be placed on the table in a team folder or on the wall, which is preferable. In figure 8.2 the chart has the team name, the team members' names, and three ways for teams to accrue points each day. You can use different categories, which might change from unit to unit but ideally not from lesson to lesson. The bonus points allow the teacher to provide additional points if the team as a whole or a member of the team makes special improvement. It is important to allow all teams to reach the same number of points each day. We recommend using three points in each category and no more than two points for bonuses. The recordkeeper is responsible for keeping the chart up to date each class session.

Using this requires teaching students their roles and responsibilities. This takes a little time but is more than made up for in each successive unit's efficiency.

Nutritionists												
Team members:												

Points Lessons	1	2	3	4	5	6	7	8	9	10	11	12	----
Following the rules													
Performing your roles													
Completing tasks													
Bonus points													
Total													

FIGURE 8.2   Sample team points log.

Summary

Few if any teachers enter the profession to be disciplinarians. Most enter the field to teach students and to see them learn their subject matter. They enjoy this aspect of teaching but complain that their time is taken up with class management. Like Mr. Barnham, they see an endless set of rules that they need to enforce and disciplinary tasks that they need to do to maintain order in the classroom. It might seem counterintuitive, but a well-organized classroom is not one with the teacher providing constant directions and information, but one where everyone knows their role. The secret to achieving this is to use a system, rehearse it, and then put it into place. Mr. Barnham's challenges could easily be mitigated by using a system. It is worth taking time in the first few lessons with a new class to lay a good foundation for the rest of your time with them.

CHAPTER 9

Building a Classroom Community

Ryan, a seventh-grader at Reunion Middle School, walks into Ms. Smith's health classroom, sits in the back, and immediately puts his head on the desk as if to signify that he intends to sleep during class. Ms. Smith notices Ryan's behavior and talks to him before the bell rings for class to begin. Ms. Smith has noticed that Ryan does not participate in most of the classroom discussion, on which Ms. Smith relies heavily in her day-to-day classroom methodology for teaching. She also believes that he does not seem particularly interested in health education and is likely to fail her class.

As Ms. Smith approaches Ryan, she asks him to raise his head off the desk and get paper out for note-taking. He complies with reluctance. When she asks him if he is tired, he responds, "Yes." She asks if he has had a good morning, and he replies, "No." She then asks him why his morning has not been good and is alarmed by his response, "Like you care." Ms. Smith begins to question what she is doing wrong in her class for a student to feel like she does not care about them.

What do we mean by this chapter's title, *Building a Classroom Community*? First, the word *building* implies that something is created. It also implies that rebuilding has to occur from time to time. A *classroom community* is dynamic, as is any social environment with several participants. The most important characteristics of building a community involve being positive, safe, caring, inclusive, and focused. A community is *positive* because having a mindset that is focused on the positive and in creating positive experiences in class is a critical foundation. A community that is *safe* means that students are comfortable to express their opinions and can take and use feedback in constructive ways. By *caring* we mean that students are in an environment characterized by mutual respect, where teachers and students engage in caring behaviors such as eye contact, kindness, and support, and where students are listened to and valued. A community is *inclusive,* indicating that the teacher uses a range of approaches to teaching that consider the diverse needs and backgrounds of all students and that the teacher has created an environment where all students feel valued and have equal access to learning. A community is *focused on learning,* indicating that students are in class for a purpose, which is to learn the content of health education. Collectively, these outcomes are not just important for learning; they are important for good health and wellness. In this chapter we focus on the rules (i.e., class policies) and on teacher and student behaviors that lead to the operationalization of these outcomes.

Why Is Building a Classroom Community Important?

In the 1950s and 1960s, if you fell while riding your bike down a neighborhood street, a neighbor on that street would likely help you up, perhaps give you some simple first aid care for your scratches, and walk with you to your parents' house. Today that is less likely to happen. Students now are confronted with this decline in social capital (Klocke and Stadtmüller 2019). Sander and Putnam (1999, p. 28) define "social capital" in this way:

> In a nutshell, it's the norms and networks of trust and reciprocity that foster collective action. More colloquially, it's the friendships, professional circles, clubs, neighborhoods, churches and alumni networks where you help the group or a fellow member because you care about and trust the group and know your action ultimately will benefit all (including you).

The networks that make up social capital provide students with an advantage in that they allow you to gain information and support and to experience trust. Conversely, the fewer networks students have, the more disadvantaged they might be (Klocke and Stadtmüller 2019). Trust is at the heart of social capital for students, who can put their trust in people (e.g., parents, teachers, friends, and coaches) and institutions (e.g., schools, sport clubs, places of worship).

As we write this book, our society is confronting social, cultural, public health, political, and economic challenges, all of which are highly interrelated and which affect students in our classes as well as ourselves. Our students, as we did, live in a different environment than past generations. Poverty, mental health, gender inequality and discrimination, disruptive pupil behavior, violent crime, living in a single-parent family, or low parent education levels can markedly increase children's chances of adverse outcomes. (See the National Center for Children in Poverty's Young Child Risk Calculator at www.nccp.org.) Though this has always been the case in modern society, it is more pronounced today and is best captured by answering the question, "Who could our students turn to for help?"

This is why a good health education curriculum should prioritize developing the skills of positive intrapersonal (e.g., self-talk) and interpersonal communication. The classroom, and the health education classroom in particular, is a key setting in helping students develop their social capital. In the school context, the improvement of social capital does not happen solely within the four walls of the school. Teachers are not psychologists, counselors, or social workers. They have neither the time nor training to deal with significant emotional challenges that confront some of their students. They do have a responsibility (1) to ensure that their classroom is positive, safe, and caring so that common challenges that students confront can be alleviated, and (2) to place students in contact with the support services and specialists in schools trained to help students.

Thinking About the Health Education Classroom as a Classroom Community

One way to think about your classroom is in terms of the Dimensions of Wellness. If a classroom were to follow the basic principles of being a "well" place, which is a foundation of health education, then the physical, social, emotional, cultural, and intellectual dimensions of the environment should be considered. These Dimensions of Wellness also align with the social and emotional learning (SEL) construct developed by Collaborative for Academic, Social, and Emotional Learning (CASEL) in 1994. SEL revolves around the ability of a student to manage positively their well-being, which includes their emotional health, while developing healthy relationships with peers and adults in the school environment, or their social health. If a classroom environment follows the same premise as SEL, it is considered a place of wellness. If an area of the classroom is not well, that area should be addressed for improvement. Similarly, when a student who is not managing their emotions well or developing healthy relationships at school, you would assess their SEL and endeavor to offer a plan for improvement.

Table 9.1 provides a description and an example of a classroom that is positive, safe, caring, and inclusive when the Dimensions of Wellness are used as a classroom guide.

TABLE 9.1   Dimensions of Wellness Framework for the Classroom

Dimension of Wellness	Definition/description	Classroom example
Physical	This describes the overall physical condition of your classroom environment.	The classroom has adequate lighting, heating, and air conditioning, and is free of hazards. Students are physically comfortable in the classroom.
Emotional	The classroom atmosphere allows for building trustworthy relationships and expressing oneself without fear.	The classroom is a place where students express their feelings about health-related matters that are important to them.
Cultural	The atmosphere is a place where no judgments based on ethnicity, religion, gender, sexual orientation, age, and customs or practices are allowed or tolerated. These things are, in fact, celebrated and expressed freely.	Students conduct project-based learning that includes cultural information regarding health behaviors and information. Students freely discuss their personal experiences in these learning exercises.
Social or interpersonal	The environment and curriculum are manipulated so that students must communicate with and rely on each other to complete tasks.	Students are placed in learning groups where health decisions must be made and goals must be set, and the consequences affect all group members equally.
Intellectual	The classroom is a place where students are learning to discover new things and solve problems.	Classroom projects require students to obtain and manipulate data in order to come to conclusions.

How to Build a Classroom Community

In this section we present a number of pedagogical strategies that you can start using tomorrow in your classes.

Address Student Needs

First, this requires getting to know who your students are. At the beginning of the year, semester, or grading term, when you are meeting students for the first time, try out some getting-to-know-you activities for all grade levels.

- Post a board with the picture and name of each student, and have them write something about themselves or a goal under their name.
- Create times when students can talk about their families and experiences.
- Have students create an artifact and add it to the room.
- Have students talk about what they see as their strengths and how they learn best.

Give Students Choices

Giving students choices allows them to exert control in their school life, which creates motivation and commitment to the lesson. It also allows students to play to their strengths. Here are some examples of choices:

- Students choose from a list you give them to help order the units of instruction you plan on teaching them. This assumes some of the units do not require other units as a prerequisite.
- Students determine with whom they sit or work on a project. Alternatively, students could give you a list of four to six students with whom they would like to sit or work. It might not always work out, and you may have to make some decisions, but if you do this two or three times in a semester, they will have worked with some of the people they nominated.
- Students determine or create criteria to judge a project or assignment.
- Students choose from a list of ways to meet a standard (e.g., project or debate). Students can demonstrate what they know in many ways, and by playing to their strengths, you will get often deeper commitment and understanding. However, when entertaining choices, be willing to say that a particular format is too easy or too hard.
- Students have a choice within a range of when an assignment or project is due.

We offer two caveats in giving students choices. The first is that it does not always work, and you need to determine how well your efforts at giving students choices worked. Consider if you actually gave them a choice, or if the instructions were clear. Do not give up after the first try; keep working on it. The second caveat is that you do not need to start off giving students a lot of choices, but by integrating more choices into your teaching, students will feel greater ownership in the lesson.

Assess Prior Knowledge

Determine what students know about what you are teaching before you teach them. You can do this in a number of ways, such as an assessment. This assessment could be a conversation, concept map, pretest, or question-and-answer session. In understanding students' prior knowledge, you can refine your instruction in a unit. This type of assessment is very helpful in determining misunderstandings about what you are going to be teaching.

Give Students Roles and Tasks in the Classroom

See the discussion in chapter 8 for examples, such as recordkeepers to take attendance in a group and organizers to hand out materials and collect work.

Be Consistent in Your Rules and Routines

See the discussion in Using a System to Organize Your Health Education Classroom in chapter 8 for examples.

Encourage Your Students to Be Positive

When John Wooden coached basketball his expectation was that his players were motivating and positive to each other. This should be an expectation in the classroom. However, students need not only a role model (i.e., you, the teacher) they also need activities and teacher-initiated activities to teach them the skills of being positive. Here are some examples of what a teacher can do to promote being positive.

- Notice and regularly reinforce students' positive interactions with each other in each lesson. You can do this initially by assigning team points in recognition of caring and positive behaviors.
- Observe students who are struggling or who have few friends. You can meet one on one with that student and set some small goals such as to sit next to a friend and asking if they would allow a friend to help them. You can seat them next to helpful students and include them in the most helpful groups as you assign tasks.
- Periodically, play some relationship-building activities that encourage sharing. The Inspired Educator (http://the-inspired-educator.com) has a number of relationship-building ideas. For example, you can use turn-and-talk pedagogy, where instead of focusing on academics, you ask students to share one good thing about the day

or something positive with their partner. You can use an exit slip that asks, "What is one kind thing you did for someone today?" Or you can use an entry slip that asks, "What is one kind thing you plan to do in this class for someone today?" Another idea is the get-to-know-you board game. Create a board with a path that has a beginning and an end. Along the path include 20 or so questions such as "What is your favorite part of the school day?" or "What is your favorite band?" The students in your class can help create the questions. Divide the class into groups of four or five students, each with a board and die; they roll the die to see which question they will answer. You can add some return-to-start spaces on the path if you wish.

- Have regular class meetings. Class meetings provide a safe environment where you can build students' confidence in discussing issues with you and their peers. One way to start this activity is for the teacher to present the issues but over time allow students to add and then drive the meeting. Start with easy-to-discuss issues, and slowly move to more demanding ones.

Model Kindness and Positivity Regularly

You can demonstrate to students that you care in many ways, including the following:

- Greet students by name as they enter the classroom.
- Plan one-on-one or small-group meetings with students during the class.
- Show interest in your students by asking about them (e.g., "How did your soccer game go last night?").
- Attend school sporting and cultural activities, and talk to your students there.
- Be aware of your students. If a student appears sad or upset, touch base with them and be someone that they can turn to for support. It may be something that you can address, or you may need to get them to a nurse or counselor.
- Finally, don't forget to be kind; to use warm, inclusive behaviors with your face, body, and words; and to smile often.

Let Students Get to Know You

Most students do not know who their teachers are. If you don't know a person, how can you trust them? In the absence of knowing their teachers, students will often have misconceptions that do not lead them to

How to Assess Your Classroom Community

Ask your students periodically in person or ask them to write their responses to questions such as the following:

- Do you feel safe in our class?
- Are students in our class kind to each other?
- Do students in our class follow the rules?
- Do you feel included by the other students?
- What is one thing I could do to improve your enjoyment of our class?
- What would you like for me to know about you at this point in time?
- Do you feel like you are learning in this class?
- Do you enjoy being in this class?

You do not need to ask all the questions at once. Rather, you could give students one minute to write responses for one or two of these questions once a week.

You can assess if your classroom community is positive, safe, caring, inclusive, and focused on learning through your own reflection on your students, or you can ask others to visit your classroom to observe you and the class. You can create a checklist that includes observations driven by questions. Following are some sample questions a teacher might ask within each dimension:

- *Physical*: Are students wearing coats to class because it is too cold in the classroom? Are all students in a seating arrangement that is conducive to learning and interaction with peers?
- *Emotional*: Have I observed all students participating? Do students tell personal stories in my classroom? Do my students ask honest, open questions about health-related topics?
- *Cultural*: Have I observed students discussing their cultural heritage during classroom activities? Do students feel comfortable discussing their religion, sexual orientation, or family customs or practices in this class?
- *Social or interpersonal*: Do students appear to like each other in this class? Do students get along during the activities that I have chosen? Do students talk to one another in appropriate ways and at appropriate times?
- *Intellectual*: Have I observed students discussing new ideas regarding health? Do students enjoy learning in this class? Do students have enough time to research and discuss their findings in this class?

view their teachers as approachable and trustworthy. To help students get to know you, you can get involved in the relationship-building games discussed earlier. Share your own experiences in ways that are developmentally appropriate and relevant during discussions. Be genuine. For example, if you do not know the answer to a student's question, tell the class you do not know but you will find out for them tomorrow. If you make a mistake, apologize for it. These events allow students to see that you are sincere and honest.

Summary

Returning to the opening vignette of Ryan in Ms. Smith's class, we would suggest to Ms. Smith that she assess her classroom both from her own perspective and from the perspective of students. She should then use the strategies in this chapter to build a classroom community that is positive, safe, caring, inclusive, and focused on learning for Ryan and his peers. In building such a community it is helpful to remember that Rome was not built in a day, and neither are classrooms. But if you start today, tomorrow you are one step closer and on the path to having a classroom that you and your students enjoy being a part of each day.

CHAPTER 10

Facilitating Classroom Discussion

Mr. Wales, a health teacher at Marion Middle School, worked hard on his goal-setting lesson for today's class. He prepared a great classroom project that focuses on healthy eating. Students will first work individually, then they will pair up to work with a partner, and then they will share with a small group. After this progression, he plans to have a full-class discussion about the healthy eating and physical activity goals the students will have created. The chairs in the classroom are organized in small groupings so that four students can face each other and talk easily, and Mr. Wales can navigate the room and have individual and group discussions as the students work on their assignments. Mr. Wales takes attendance as the students enter the room and instructs them to begin working on their individual assignment that was on the smartboard: "Think: What is one goal you will set for healthy eating this week?" After letting the students work on their assignment individually for a few minutes, he then tells them to pair up with someone in their group and move to the second part of the assignment, which he reveals on the smartboard: "Pair: With your partner, discuss your goal." After several minutes, Mr. Wales notices that the room is exceptionally quiet. He observes a few students whispering together and decides to prompt all students to begin working in their groups on the third part of the assignment. He reveals on the smartboard the next part: "Share: Discuss your goal with your group." After several minutes, Mr. Wales realizes that the students are not engaging with each other. As he moves around the room, students engage with him, but they are not working on the assignment together. Many of them seem to be answering the initial question listed on the smartboard, but they are not interacting and discussing their goals as the next steps of the project prompted them to do. Mr. Wales is stumped at figuring out how to get the students to discuss the lesson's content with each other.

What Is a Classroom Discussion?

A classroom discussion is a sustained exchange between and among teachers and their students with the purpose of developing students' capabilities or skills and of expanding students' understanding—both shared and individual—of a specific concept or instructional goal. Classroom discussions are characterized by high-quality and high quantities of student talk. Teachers must ensure that discussions are built upon and revolve around both students' contributions and the content at hand. In a discussion, the teacher's role is to question students; take up, revoice, and press students' ideas; structure and steer the conversation toward the learning goals; enable students to respond to one another's ideas by stepping back to listen; moderate and facilitate students' interactions; ensure that the content under discussion is represented accurately; and bring the discussion to a meaningful close (Witherspoon, Sykes, and Bell 2016, p. 6).

A classroom discussion involves teamwork. The teacher and students are dependent on each other to make discussion work: "In instructionally productive discussions, the teacher and a wide range of students contribute orally, listen actively, and respond to and learn from others' contributions" (Grossman 2018, p. 185). Teachers should use class discussion for three reasons:

1. *Discussions in class increase student connection and engagement with the content.* Health lessons should not be dominated by lectures. Including discussions in lessons allows students to delve deeper into the content and be reflective as they engage in discussion. It also allows students to see and understand different perspectives on the topic from their peers such as individuals' risks in a public health crisis such as the COVID-19 pandemic or the extent to which some individuals will tolerate being overweight.

2. *Discussions in class allow the teacher both to reinforce student positions and to correct misunderstandings.* Student discussion allows teachers to see students' progress in understanding and to shape student understanding as they answer questions and discuss positions with their peers and teacher.

3. *Discussions in class develop students' decision-making and interpersonal skills.* Frequent discussions provide opportunities for students to state their positions, listen to the positions of others without interrupting, speak with increasing confidence and assertiveness, be empathic with other positions or peers, negotiate, problem-solve, and be a contributing member of a team. All of these are real-world functional skills and are part of the National Health Education Standards (NHES).

General Principles for Discussions

General principles are guidelines you can use when preparing for and conducting discussions. You do not need to do all of these things, but you should consider them. Doing them initially will develop purposely constructed lessons. Over time they will likely become teaching habits.

Prepare Prior to the Class

Following these three steps prior to teaching will be helpful.

Step 1: Create Your Discussion Questions

While planning for the health lesson, teachers must not only plan for the active learning strategy of discussion, but they must plan the discussion itself. The first step when planning for discussion is to determine your discussion questions. In considering the following four points, the teacher can determine if the questions create dependence and trust and if there is a logical sequence in questioning.

1. Are these questions related to the assessment for today's lesson?
2. Do students have to ask a question of their peers or teacher in order to move to the next learning segment or learn more information?
3. Will all students feel safe when answering these questions?
4. Will all students feel safe sharing their answers with their peers or teacher?

If Mr. Wales had answered these questions, he would have been able to address the mistake he made while determining his questions. The question, "What is one goal you will set for healthy eating this week?" does not create dependence on the peers or teacher. If Mr. Wales would follow it up by asking how their goal is similar to and different from their partner's in the Pair activity, this would create dependence. In order for students to answer this question, they would have to discuss each other's goals from the Think activity.

Step 2: Determine Which Method Will Work Best for Facilitating the Questions

While discussion is a great active learning strategy, a teacher can perform the activity in the classroom in many ways. From whole-class discussion to small groups, from random partners to selected partners, from open-ended to scripted questions, discussion can happen in many forms. It is important to determine which method works for the particular lesson that is being taught that day. Discussion often takes up ample class time, so if the teacher has a lot of material to get through then a short discussion is important. If the topic at hand is timely and relevant and class time is not as important as the discussion topic, a lengthier discussion may be warranted. In each scenario the number of questions to be processed may not be proportionate to the time needed. For example, if there has been a death in the school, a class discussion to allow students to express their feelings may be necessary. An entire class period may be set aside for this discussion, with only one or two questions that are posed to the group of students.

Step 3: Facilitate the Questions

How will you present the questions to your students? Mr. Wales used the smartboard. This facilitation method did work for him. Students read it and were answering the initial question. The breakdown for Mr. Wales was in step 1; he started out with the wrong questions. He planned well for steps 2 and 3. The teacher must determine the best way to present the questions so that students will want to answer them and then discuss with their peers and the teacher.

Before the discussion starts, ask students to take several minutes to write down everything they know about the topic of the discussion, which will prime them for the discussion. This is an active learning activity called individual brainstorming.

What to Do During Discussion

Anything can happen in a class discussion. Students can make inappropriate comments, get in arguments, cry, or be silent. Many teachers choose not to engage in discussion because of these unknown factors. However, discussion can be a very informative experience for teachers. It is during discussion that teachers can get to know their students on a deeper level and learn things about their students that they might not otherwise know. When students feel safe and trust their teacher and the classroom environment, they often open up about things that are discussed only in health class. It is important that teachers monitor and take note of the answers, perhaps in a private journal or note-taking system so that a record is kept. This will allow you to see patterns, such as abuse or possible mental and emotional health issues, that need to be addressed by referral to the school nurse or counselor. The recordkeeping should include the student's name, date, time, and what was said. This can be looked back upon if a situation becomes more serious and the authorities become involved.

It is also important to monitor student behavior during discussions. Some students may be dealing with anger management issues or depression or other emotional issues, which can be triggered during discussions. Students may be more likely to lash out at peers or teachers during discussions. The teacher must consider this in step 1 while creating the discussion questions. The best way to prevent classroom disruptions is planning. Peer interactions might also play a role in how students behave during discussions. If certain peers do not get along, it is important to put them in different groups so that conflict does not escalate. If other peers are intimidated by or shy around other peers, they may not participate in the discussion. Trying to determine which students would be successful in discussing together is the job of the teacher. This is important to consider during the planning of the lesson and will help nurture trust with students and teachers. Here are some other tips to follow:

- Use students' names, and consider naming groups.
- Each student should have an opportunity to speak.
- Encourage students to look at and talk to each other rather than to just look and talk to you. Too often discussions take the format of a dialogue between the teacher and a series of students.
- If possible, make the class space more conducive to discussion. Arrange seats in a circle or in a manner that enables students to see each other easily. Do not let students sit in seats that are outside this discussion space.
- After asking a question, wait at least eight to ten seconds before calling on someone to answer it; measure the time by counting silently to yourself. Otherwise, you signal they need only wait a few seconds for the "right" answer to discussion questions from you.

Posing Discussion Questions

Here are some kinds of questions that will elicit more student discussion.

- Ask questions that encourage responses from several people (e.g., "What do the rest of you think about that?").
- Use phrasing that implies that the students are a learning community (e.g., "Are we in agreement?" or "Do we have any differences of opinion?").
- Ask a mix of questions, including questions that ask students to
  - recall specific information,
  - describe topics and phenomena,

- apply abstract concepts to concrete situations,
- connect the general with the specific,
- combine topics or concepts to form new topics or concepts, and
- evaluate information.

- Avoid yes-and-no questions or questions that can be answered in one word (e.g., "Is X true?"). Open-ended questions elicit student thought (e.g., "In what way has X affected Y?").

- Avoid asking, "Are there any questions?" This implies you have finished talking about a topic. Sensing that you have said your piece, students may only ask questions about minor points of clarification or will simply hope that rereading the textbook will answer their questions. Consider asking instead, "Is there anything that is unclear or needs further clarification?"

- Avoid dissertation questions. If you want your students to entertain broad questions, break the question down into smaller queries that students are more able to address.

Dignify Your Students

Students are more likely to participate in discussion if they feel valued by the teacher, if they feel safe in speaking, and if they feel heard. Here are a number of strategies that help build dignity among students.

- Avoid a style of questioning that is designed to punish inattentive or lazy students.

- Treat your students like experts. If a student makes a good comment, refer back to that comment in subsequent discussions (e.g., "Do you recall what Henry said last week? How does this new information confirm or deny his conclusion?").

- Allow a student to pass on a question, but come back to them later in class.

- Admit when you make a mistake in class. Similarly, if a student asks you a question to which you do not know the answer, promise to research the question after class or to provide students with appropriate resources to find the answer themselves.

- Keep the discussion focused because you want to respect the students' time.

- State the discussion topic at the beginning of the class because you want students to know and be prepared for the discussion.

- Periodically summarize the main themes or points brought out in discussion to keep students focused on the key elements of the discussion. Consider writing these main themes or points on the board or in the class digital notes.

End Discussion Smoothly

- Review the main points of the discussion or ask a student, whom you notified previously, to review the main points.

- At the end of the discussion, allow students to write down any conclusions or lingering questions they have. Perhaps ask them how the discussion affected their views on a topic or their understanding of a concept. Ask several students to share their responses.

- Point out how the day's discussion will tie in with the next discussion.

Types of Discussion Formats

The following discussion formats are presented with the permission of Jennifer Gonzalez. For more details on any of these formats see www.cultofpedagogy.com.

Gallery Walk

This is also known as chat stations or the carousel activity. Stations or posters are set up around the classroom, on the walls or on tables. Small groups of students travel from station to station together, performing some kind of task or responding to a prompt, either of which will result in a conversation.

Philosophical Chairs

This is also known as values continuum, forced debate, physical barometer, or this or that. A statement that has two possible responses—agree or disagree—is read out loud. Depending on whether they agree or disagree with this statement, students move to one side of the room or the other. From that spot, students take turns defending their positions.

Pinwheel Discussion

Students are divided into four groups. Three of these groups are assigned to represent specific points of view. Members of the fourth group are designated as "provocateurs," tasked with making sure the discussion keeps going and stays challenging. One person from each group (the "speaker") sits in a desk facing speakers from the other groups, so they form a square in the center of the room. Behind each speaker, the remaining group members are seated: two right behind the speaker, then three behind them, and so on, forming a kind of triangle. From above, this would look like a pinwheel. The four speakers introduce and discuss questions they prepared ahead of time (this preparation is done with their groups). After some time passes, new students rotate from the seats behind the speaker into the center seats and continue the conversation.

Socratic Seminar

This is also known as Socratic circles. Students prepare by reading a text or group of texts and writing some higher-order discussion questions about the text. On seminar day, students sit in a circle, and an introductory, open-ended question is posed by the teacher or student discussion leader. From there, students continue the conversation, prompting one another to support their claims with textual evidence. There is no particular order to how students speak, but they are encouraged to respectfully share the floor with others. Discussion is meant to happen naturally, and students do not need to raise their hands to speak. The overview of Socratic Seminar from the website Facing History and Ourselves provides a list of appropriate questions, plus more information about how to prepare for a seminar (www.facinghistory.org).

Affinity Mapping

This is also known as affinity diagramming. Give students a broad question or problem that is likely to result in lots of different ideas, such as "What were the impacts of the Great Depression?" or "What literary works should every person read?" Have students generate responses by writing ideas on Post-it notes (one idea per note) and placing them in no particular arrangement on a wall, whiteboard, or chart paper. Once lots of ideas have been generated, have students begin grouping them into similar categories, then label the categories and discuss why the ideas fit within them, how the categories relate to one another, and so on.

Concentric Circles

This is also known as speed dating. Students form two circles, one inside circle and one outside circle. Each student on the inside is paired with a student on the outside; they face each other. The teacher poses a question to the whole group, and pairs discuss their responses with each other, then the teacher signals students to rotate. Students on the outside circle move one space to the right so they are standing (or sitting) in front of a new person. Now the teacher poses a new question, and the process is repeated.

Conver-Stations

This is a small-group discussion strategy that gives students exposure to more of their peers' ideas and prevents the stagnation that can occur when a group does not happen to have the right chemistry. Students are placed into a few groups of four to six students each and are given a discussion question to talk about. After sufficient time has passed for the discussion to develop, one or two students from each group rotate to a different group, while the other group members remain where they are. Once in their new group, they will discuss a different but related question, and they may also share some of the key points from their last group's conversation. For the next rotation, students who have not rotated before may be chosen to move, resulting in groups that are continually evolving. Teachers may give students numbers and call out the numbers that are supposed to move on their prompt.

Fishbowl

Two students sit facing each other in the center of the room; the remaining students sit in a circle around them. The two central students have a conversation based on a predetermined topic and often using specific skills the class is practicing (e.g., asking follow-up questions, paraphrasing, or elaborating on another person's point). Students on the outside observe, take notes, or perform some other discussion-related task assigned by the teacher.

Hot Seat

One student assumes the role of a book character, significant figure in history, or concept (e.g., a tornado, a vaccine, or Henrietta Lacks). Sitting in front of the rest of the class, the student responds to classmates' questions while staying in character in that role.

Snowball Discussion

This is also known as pyramid discussion. Students begin in pairs, responding to a discussion question only with a single partner. After each person has had a chance to share their ideas, the pair joins another pair, creating a group of four. Pairs share their ideas with the pair they just joined. Next, groups of four join together to form groups of eight, and so on, until the whole class is joined up in one large discussion. (This is similar to the Think, Pair, Share activity discussed earlier in this chapter, except the pairing continues.)

Ongoing Discussion Strategies

Whereas the other formats in this list have a distinct shape—specific *activities* you do with students—the strategies in this section are more like plug-ins, working discussion into other instructional activities and improving the quality and reach of existing conversations.

Talk Moves

This is also known as accountable talk. Talk moves are sentence frames you supply to your students that help them express ideas and interact with one another in respectful, academically appropriate ways. From kindergarten all the way through college, students can benefit from explicit instruction in the skills of summarizing another person's argument before presenting an alternate view, asking clarifying questions, and expressing agreement or partial agreement with the stance of another participant. Talk moves can be incorporated into any of the other discussion formats listed here. This strategy directly aligns with Standard 4 of NHES on communication and will help you address lesson objectives for this standard.

Teach-OK

This is a peer teaching strategy that begins with the teacher spending a few minutes introducing a concept to the class. Next, the teacher says, *"Teach!"* the class responds with *"OK!"* and pairs of students take turns reteaching the concept to each other. It is a bit like think-pair-share (see the next section), but it's faster paced, it focuses more on reteaching than general sharing, and students are encouraged to use gestures to animate their discussion.

Think-Pair-Share

An oldie but a goodie, think-pair-share can be used any time you want to plug interactivity into a lesson: Simply have students *think* about their response to a question, form a *pair* with another person, discuss their response, then *share* it with the larger group. This strategy has so many uses and can be more powerful than it is given credit for.

TQE (Thoughts, Questions, and Epiphanies) Method

This protocol has students come up with their own **thoughts**, lingering **questions**, and **epiphanies** from an assigned reading. Teachers who have used this method say it has generated some of the richest conversations they have ever heard from students.

Ongoing Conversations

This strategy places students into one-on-one conversations, getting them to learn each other's names better and create a track record of what they talked about. This strategy is excellent for classes in which you want to help students get more comfortable with each other.

Challenges in Discussions

A teacher must have an understanding of why students under- or over-contribute in order to match a strategy to that particular student's needs. Note that not all of the following suggestions work with all students.

Students Who Do Not Contribute

A student may not contribute for many reasons, including introversion, shyness, low proficiency in speaking English because it is their second language, cultural differences, or punishing experiences in the past with engaging in discussions. Following are some strategies to employ:

- A first step is to talk with students to find out their hesitance in discussions. Share with them your understanding and provide them with specific ways to engage in a discussion, such as writing down some thoughts before contributing or having them preplan what they want to say. You can help them do this by adding more information in the syllabus or providing a handout in the prior lesson relative to the topics being discussed.
- Create an expectation that everyone will share their views.
- Praise students for sharing.
- Rotate team members to share information with the class or lead the discussion.

- Because what happens in a class occurs in a fishbowl and everyone knows what is going on, consider recruiting students in a group to be supportive of students who are not contributing. Be sure to share how they could be supportive such as praise, smiling, and clapping or finger snapping.

Students Who Contribute More Than Appropriate

One approach is to work with the student on listening. Role-playing can help with this. This can be done as a class without identifying students, such as the following partner activities:

- Students listen and then tell their partner what they heard. The pair then switches roles.
- Active listening games, many of which can be found online.
- Assign the student who overcontributes the role of making sure everyone in the group speaks.

Students Who Are Disruptive in the Discussion

Make the group responsible for controlling unproductive antagonists by structuring a group response (e.g., articulate the student's position, perhaps on the chalkboard) and asking for a response from the student who is disrupting.

Summary

Classroom discussions increase student connection and engagement with the content, allow teachers both to determine student understanding and to correct misunderstandings, and strengthen student decision-making and communication and interpersonal skills. They add depth and quality to understanding the content of the lesson. If Mr. Wales had prepared discussion questions and used any of the strategies discussed in this chapter, he might have more successfully met his objectives for the lesson and better connected with his students.

CHAPTER 11

Providing Feedback to Students

Mrs. Witt has given a performance task to be completed over the next few days. Students have been asked to track their food and drink for 48 hours, enter the data into a fitness app that analyzes the data, and write an assessment of their nutrition, describing things that are going well and things that need improvement. In the following classes she provides feedback to the class and individual students as they ask questions about how to complete the assignments. As she started to grade the assignment, she quickly realized that many students had not done the assignment correctly. Mrs. Witt felt that she had described the task well. Since so many students seemed to have missed key elements of the assignment, she considered if the problem might have been the feedback. The next day she talked to her class about the feedback. Her students said that sometimes the feedback was confusing or not related to the problem that they were dealing with.

Feedback has been debated for at least a century in the educational world, and it is one of the most misunderstood teaching skills. Here are a few questions you might consider:

- Is positive or negative feedback better?
- How timely does it need to be?
- How detailed does it need to be?
- Is specific or general feedback better, or is there some value to both?
- Should teachers provide feedback all the time, some of the time, or not at all?
- Is it feedback if the teacher says something, but it doesn't result in the behavior the teacher wants?
- Is feedback to be viewed discretely or part of a longer-term strategy to support learning?
- Does feedback advance student learning?

In any search of the literature, you can probably find a wide variety of views. For us, the bottom line is that feedback is necessary and should result in improved learning outcomes, such as improvement in student understanding, knowledge, and performance.

Feedback has been proven to increase learning and improve student outcomes (Hattie and Timperley 2007). Feedback also clarifies goals, enhances commitment, and increases student effort and task persistence (Hattie and Timperley 2007). When feedback is given correctly, it guides students forward in their understanding and performance of content and keeps them on track to achieve the goals of the lesson or unit of instruction. Feedback also lets students know that the instructor cares enough about them and their learning to help them, and this in turn creates commitment and engagement from students. In this chapter we first address some common evidence-based rules for giving feedback and then discuss some systems of feedback and how to create a culture of feedback.

Ground Rules for Providing Feedback

Here are some important ideas to consider when giving feedback.

Feedback Should Be Specific

Statements such as "That needs improvement" or "Keep thinking" do not provide students with clear information on what to do to improve. Moreover, feedback that is not specific may make students feel the feedback is useless or the teacher is uncaring, which might affect student effort and learning. Feedback is significantly more effective when it provides details of how to improve the answer or performance rather than simply indicating whether the student's work is correct or not. However, feedback does not always need to be directive (e.g., "Don't forget to provide a description of what happens when . . . " or "I see this sentence has commas, but the next one doesn't seem to have any"). It can also promote critical thinking (e.g., "Have you considered X?" "What topics connected to this discussion did you not talk about?" "What do we already know about X?" "What would happen if . . . ?" "Can you think of an example?").

Feedback Should Be Aligned With the Goal and Subtask

Subtasks reflect goals that everyone in the class, both teacher and students, knows are to be achieved. An example of a goal in health education is a class assignment prompt such as, "We are going to do a project where we use recycled materials to create something useful or beautiful and try to persuade others to recycle." Feedback should be aligned with the goal or subtasks of the goal. This seems obvious because, for example, you do not want to provide feedback on communicable diseases when the lesson is about noncommunicable diseases. But very often teachers have a tendency to go on a tangent to provide information that is not relevant to the task. A funny example of this is telling someone how rubber is made when all they wanted to know was how to change a tire. The message here is that feedback must be purposeful and focused.

Feedback Should Be Given in a Timely Manner

Research shows that most often feedback that is provided immediately results in better learning. If you wait too long to give feedback, the moment is lost, and students might not connect the feedback with their efforts. Timely means that the students receive feedback when they can use it. If you are in the middle of class management and a student asks for feedback on a project, it will have to wait until you resolve the management issue. Feedback given a lesson or a week after a question was asked is typically not as effective as feedback given in the lesson in which the query was raised.

Feedback Comes in Different Forms

Most of the feedback discussed here is called formative feedback. This means that it happens while learning is occurring and not when the project is finished. Feedback provided at the end of the project is called summative feedback and is often tied to evaluation of the project or task. Feedback can be given verbally, nonverbally, or in written form. However, the function of feedback is important. Some feedback functions to keep students working, which often takes the form of praise, such as "Keep up the good work." Some feedback prompts or reminds students, such as "Don't forget to provide an example." Some feedback is corrective, such as "You need to place the diagram on the left," or "Add more information about the COVID-19 pandemic here." Some feedback, as we have already discussed, serves to stimulate critical thinking in the form of questions, such as "What are your thoughts about . . .?" "How do you think we can improve this situation?" or "What do you suggest can be done?"

Feedback Systems

Teachers spend all day providing feedback to their students. That will likely never change, but teachers can involve students in self and peer feedback in ways that create deeper learning experiences and involve the class in supporting the goal of learning. In this section we discuss some feedback systems that teachers can use routinely in class.

Feedback Loops

A feedback loop consists of students doing work, comparing their work to a rubric or a set of criteria, and then making edits. Finally, students reflect on the edits and what they have learned about the content and the process of editing. It is designed to advance students toward higher levels of academic achievement and to engage them more deeply in learning the content. For feedback loops to be effective, they must

- be purposeful and goal-focused,
- be specific and nonevaluative,
- allow for correction, and
- include self-reflection.

Figure 11.1 provides an example of a feedback loop that could be used for a component of a project or a task. In this example, Juan evaluates his own work, makes edits, then shares his work with a peer or peers, who provide feedback to him. He then makes edits again. At the end of the process Juan considers what he has learned about the content, and he shares that with the class or the teacher. The teacher could have used several cycles of feedback and edits. In this example self and peer feedback could also involve teacher feedback.

Speed Feedback

This is the academic version of speed dating. Typically, we use two and three cycles of feedback. The feedback is done in pairs, and students rotate to new students. In class each table has four or five students. Each student is assigned a color for the term. The teacher pairs up two colors, and that is who each student works with. Each student reads their partner's work or listens to the partner discuss their idea. Then the reader or listener has 30 seconds to provide feedback. If it is written work, the two students read their work for one minute and then take 30 seconds each

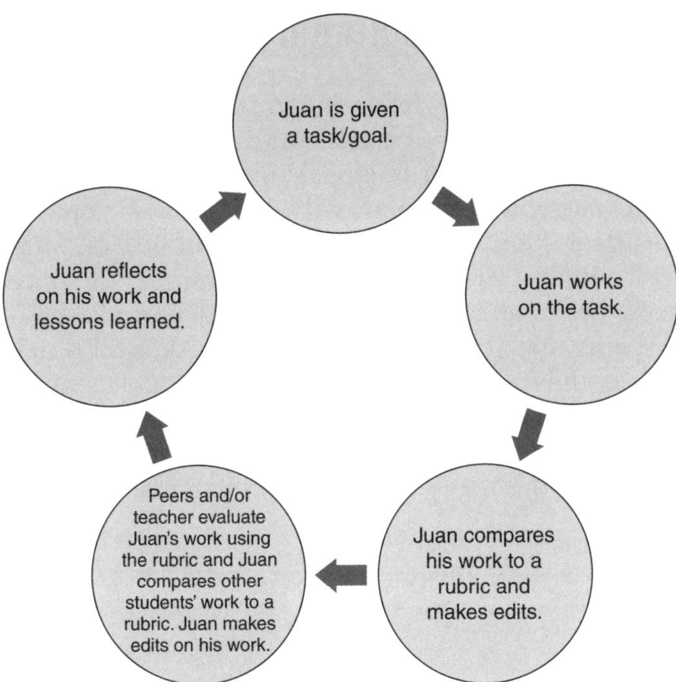

FIGURE 11.1   An example of a feedback loop.

to provide feedback. (*Note*: In this case, the amount of writing needs to be limited to what most students can read in one minute.) If students are sharing ideas, offer 30 seconds to the partner first sharing ideas and 30 seconds of feedback, then switch students. Be sure that the person receiving feedback takes notes on what to change.

Microconferences

Microconferences take one to two minutes to do, present one-on-one opportunities to individualize instruction and feedback, fix misconceptions, and build relationships between the teacher and the student. First, read all the students' work, and add sticky notes to each one with your feedback or write on the work itself. Meet with the students to talk through the feedback and give them time to ask questions. If you meet with 10 students, for example, the entire process takes 20 minutes; it will not take more than a day or so to get through the entire class. However, the class will need to have a project to work on during this time rather than sitting and waiting for their turn.

Summary

In health education, the goal is for students to engage in behaviors that affect their health and life positively and to influence others to do the same along the way. Without feedback, students will not know if they are on a path that will help them with the behavior changes that are necessary to affect their health and the health of others. After reflecting more on her feedback, Mrs. Witt has found a number of approaches that she can use in her health classroom. She understands the importance of feedback being specific, aligned with the task, and timely. She also realizes that she has a number of ways to provide feedback and that she can use feedback to serve different functions. She was most excited to consider that she could use systems of feedback not just to improve student learning and engagement, but to aid in her efforts to provide timely feedback.

CHAPTER 12

Adapting Teaching to Meet the Needs of Students

Mr. Haun is looking forward to his ninth-grade health class this year. The fall semester is exciting for him because each year he has a new group of students who come from the local middle schools, and he enjoys getting to know them, their culture, abilities, life experiences, learning histories, and preferences. He also enjoys learning about their health education knowledge and skill acquisition that they have had up until this point in their K-12 careers. As Mr. Haun begins teaching, he realizes that his students differ in terms of their prior knowledge and experiences and their learning styles. He also realizes that their command of English differs because for some English is a second language. It becomes clear to him that he needs to work with students differently to meet their diverse needs.

Addressing the diverse educational needs of individual students in today's classrooms is a challenging task for teachers to master. The term *adaptive teaching* means that a teacher is responsive to the needs of students. In short, it is a commitment to meet all students where they are. This can occur in planning and in practice. In planning it occurs as teachers reflect on what they know about their students, and in practice it occurs in the operationalization of their teaching plan. Many classrooms operate with a one-size-fits-all approach in terms of structure and curriculum, with little accommodation of the learning needs, cultural backgrounds, and individual interests of students. In contrast, an adaptive teacher varies the content and pedagogy by considering students' learning needs, cultural-linguistic backgrounds, and demonstrated knowledge. This does not mean 30 different activities or approaches for 30 students in a classroom.

How to Determine Where Students Are Relative to Your Content

You can get to know your students in two ways. First, you learn who they are as people and, second, you determine their knowledge of health education and academic skill set.

Who Are Your Students?

The sidebar Writing Prompts for Students to Help Teachers Get to Know Them presents a series of writing prompts in different formats that will help you gather information to better understand your students. Some of the prompts ask for the same information but in a different way. Select the prompts that reflect what you want to know, and modify the language of these prompts to fit your grade level. You do not have to present these to students all at once or even in the first week you are with them, nor do you need to use all of these questions or their headings. You could ask students to complete three to five questions during several class periods, perhaps while attendance is being taken. We recommend

Writing Prompts for Students to Help Teachers Get to Know Them

Goals

- What are your career goals?
- What are your educational goals after high school?
- What college would you like to attend?
- What do you see yourself doing in the next five years?

Family and Home Environment

- How many brothers and sisters do you have?
- Do you take the bus to school?
- Do you bring your own lunch to school?
- What language do you speak at home?
- Whom do you know, other than a teacher, who has gone to college?

Personal Information

- Who are your friends in this class?
- What are you are most proud of?
- What do you enjoy doing in your free time?
- What extracurricular activities are you involved in?
- What are your hobbies?

- What are your favorite things to do when you are not in school?
- Tell me about what you did this summer.
- Describe one thing that makes you feel a sense of accomplishment. Explain why.
- What is one thing you wish I knew about you?
- What is your biggest dream in life?
- What is one thing you wish you could change about our school? Why?
- What is one thing that you worry about?
- What is the best book you have ever read? Why did you like it?
- If you could go anywhere, where would you go?
- You learn the most when the teacher . . .
- What can you do to learn the most?
- What is your ideal job?
- What is one thing that makes you feel happy?
- Who is someone you consider a friend? What do you like most about him or her?
- Describe something that annoys you.
- Who is someone you consider a hero in your life? Why?
- If you could live anywhere, where would you live? Why?
- What is one of your favorite [insert holiday] traditions?
- What is your religious background?
- What are three adjectives others might use to describe you?

School

- What is your favorite thing about school?
- What is your least favorite thing about school?
- What was your favorite class last year? Why?
- Why did you enroll in this class?
- What school clubs and organizations do you belong to?
- What school sports are you involved with?
- What extracurricular activities (sports, band, student council, etc.) do you want to participate in this year?

Teacher and Class

- What is one thing you would really like to know about [teacher name]?
- What is the most important thing I need to do as a teacher to help you succeed in our class?
- What is one thing you wish you could change about this class? Why?

writing the questions on sheets of paper with space for the students to write. When they are finished you can clip them together to have a record of each student. Alternatively, you could create a file as shown in table 12.1 that contains some essential information you have collected from both students and their school records. It is important to remember that students do not need to divulge any information they are not comfortable sharing. This message must be communicated so they do not feel pressured to disclose things that they feel are too personal. Teachers must also be aware, however, that students may feel comfortable sharing very personal and private information and that these things must be kept confidential unless you have concerns of something improper or illegal happening in the home or with peers. The point of the prompts is to get to know your students to determine where students are in relationship to your class as a whole and the health content you are teaching.

What Are Your Students' Knowledge of Health Education and Academic Skill Sets?

You have access to your students' academic records, which should include information about their reading levels. You will also need to have access to the records of those students who have individualized education

TABLE 12.1 An Example of Student Records

Name	Family	Friends	Academics	Allergies	Health	Culture	IEP	Interests
Juan K.	Parents divorced. Both parents remarried: mom/husband (Sofia/José) father/wife (Luis/Joanne)	Weidong, Booker, and Robert	Reading age test scores: 74%	None	Good	Grandparents from New Mexico. Mexican; Spanish is often spoken at home.	Yes—mild autism	Soccer, science, and running
Jillian B.	Parents	Julie, Susan, and Bobbie	Reading age test scores: 81%	Peanuts	Asthma	Family from Ohio	No	Ballet and dogs
Kwame W.	Lives with father (Sam) and grandmother (Ada)	Trevor, Cornell, and Booker	Reading age test scores: 56%	None	Good	Born in Ohio. Family from South Carolina	No	Basketball

programs (IEPs). An IEP is a written document that is developed for each student who is eligible for special education. If a student with an IEP is in your class, you will have helped develop it or will review it each year.

Additionally, at the start of each unit you could offer a pretest to determine what knowledge your students have acquired about health education. See chapter 7 for ideas on how to do this.

What to Do Once You Have Determined Where Students Are Relative to Your Content

There are many different yet appropriate ways that students' needs can be accommodated. In this section we present some common strategies to do so. Specifically, we discuss how to adapt instruction in the health education classroom in such a way that students can learn the health knowledge and skills that will affect them for life.

Flexible Grouping

Tomlinson and Moon (2013) identify flexible grouping as an element of instruction that is well suited for the health education classroom and that can be easily adapted for the diverse learner. This strategy ensures that students get to work with a variety of peers in their class, regularly and frequently. We believe students should work with each other at least on a weekly basis, but even more frequently is better. Peer work should be a regular expectation in a health education classroom. This provides the opportunity for students to work with peers who learn similarly and differently, who share the same and different interests, and who approach the task in the same or a different style. It is also important that sometimes the groups are randomly created, sometimes teacher selected, and sometimes peer designed. These opportunities allow for students to learn and acknowledge their own strengths and needs and those of their peers. This is important in health education, a topic in which strengths and needs can be life-enhancing or life-threatening.

Key to flexible grouping is that it must be planned. If it is not planned for, the opportunities will not occur. Too many things will draw the teacher away from groups (e.g., a noisy classroom or students who do not get along) if no purposeful plan is in place for flexible grouping.

We suggest using the framework from chapters 2 through 4 (big ideas, enduring understandings, and essential questions) to determine what you will teach and including how you will choose your flexible grouping during your planning. This will force you to think ahead about how you will create groups and what the purposes of the groups are for the lessons.

The sidebar Tobacco Unit provides an example of this planning outcome. The first section shows the outcome of the planning process described in chapters 2 through 4. The next section shows how the essential questions are addressed in the lessons. The last section shows the purposeful planning of flexible grouping. Note that this is a simplified example to show how the connections are made.

Tobacco Unit

	Lesson 1	Lesson 2	Lesson 3	Lesson 4
Health Content	Effect on the lungs	Why do people smoke?	Helping others refuse and/or quit	Vaping—don't start a bad habit
Health Skill	Accessing valid health information	Analyzing influences	Advocacy	Decision-making
Grouping strategy	Teacher created, mixed technology skills	Random groups, peer created	Teacher created, same abilities	No groups

The point of planning for flexible grouping is that you allow the students to have different opportunities to find ways to learn from each other. This adaptation will create a learning atmosphere that ensures that all students, instead of a select few students, feel as though their strengths and needs are being addressed by their teacher.

Project-Based Learning

The next strategy that will increase adaptation in the health education classroom is project-based learning (PBL). The Buck Institute for Education's PBLWorks initiative (www.pblworks.org) describes PBL as "a teaching method in which students learn by actively engaging in real-world and personally meaningful projects." This method works to adapt instruction to student learning by having students choose projects based on their own interests and abilities, provides students ample time to work on the project (from one week to an entire semester), gives students support to complete the project, and then has students present the outcome of their project. By presenting their project, they demonstrate how they have addressed a complex, real-world problem while learning content, in our case health education content and skills. The PBLWorks initiative promotes a Gold Standard model that is based on research and aligns with the High Quality PBL framework (https://hqpbl.org/). This framework suggests that high-quality PBL must include the following six student-centered criteria: intellectual challenge and accomplishment, authenticity, public product, collaboration, project management, and reflection. Table 12.2 provides an overview of the six criteria for using PBL in health education. This example project is centered on mental and emotional health and focuses on the question "How can our school reduce bullying?" This example

TABLE 12.2 An Overview of a PBL Project in Health

Intellectual challenge and accomplishment	• Students are given one month to complete the project. • Students will investigate bullying in their school. They will learn about policies, cases reported, discipline procedures, and prevention activities. • They will also investigate the health education curriculum to determine how health education can help with this problem.
Authenticity	• Students will use interviewing techniques with school and community personnel and students to find out real-world information about bullying. • They will use library and computer resources to conduct research to find statistics on bullying. • They will determine the direction they would like their project to focus on as they obtain answers to their questions.
Public product	• First, students will present their findings to their classmates, who will give them feedback. • Next, they will present it to their school administration. • If time permits, they will present it to their school board and the public.
Collaboration	• Students will work together in groups of three. They will investigate like reporters, by conducting interviews and doing research, and work on their final product presentation. • They might also work with the district's bullying task force.
Project management	• Students will use project management skills. For example, but not limited to, they will create an outline of the project tasks (e.g., interview the principal, call the chair of the bullying task force), create a timeline for work to be completed, and delegate work to particular people.
Reflection	• Students will keep a journal to reflect on the process of investigating bullying in their school. • They will have weekly team meetings to critique each other's findings and make any necessary changes before they proceed to the next week's assignments.

is not exhaustive of the entire project; rather it provides an idea from which to gain an understanding of high-quality PBL.

As you teach health education content and skills and guide students through their learning, we recommend using the seven project-based teaching practices of Gold Standard PBL (see www.pblworks.org). These practices will ensure that you adapt instruction so that all students can perform the indicators of the National Health Education Standards according to their age and developmental level. The seven practices are

1. design and plan,
2. align to standards,
3. build the culture,
4. manage activities,
5. scaffold student learning,
6. assess student learning, and
7. engage and coach.

Kokotsaki, Menzies, and Wiggins (2016, p. 267) describe "project-based learning (PBL) [as] an active student-centered form of instruction which is characterized by students' autonomy, constructive investigations, goal-setting, collaboration, communication and reflection within real-world practices." They discuss six recommendations based on a literature review that will help PBL to be successful in your classroom: student support; teacher support; effective group work; balancing didactic instruction with independent inquiry method; assessment emphasis on reflection and on self and peer evaluation; and student choice and autonomy. We provide an overview of each in the following sections but focus on those that directly help to adapt instruction to meet students' needs, in particular, balancing didactic instruction with independent inquiry and student choice and autonomy.

Student Support

Students in the health classroom need to be supported and guided as they develop their health projects. They need to be guided in their time spent on tasks, such as research and development, and in managing their academic behaviors (e.g., organization, using the computer safely, etc.). Additionally, they need to have ample time and resources to complete the projects.

Teacher Support

Health teachers need the support of their administrators and colleagues to continue to grow in their field. This support, which can take the form of money for attending professional health teacher conferences and resources for teaching health in their classrooms, is necessary in order for teachers to have robust ideas for PBL and to incorporate it successfully.

Effective Group Work

As discussed earlier, group planning and group work instruction is an important part of planning an effective health project in which all students have an equal opportunity to learn. Health teachers must ensure that all members of the group are able and willing to participate in the project.

Balancing Didactic Instruction With Independent Inquiry

Didactic health instruction is instruction given directly to students to impart health knowledge and skills; generally, it is teacher-centered. Independent inquiry in health education occurs when students work on a health project independently with minimal teacher guidance; generally, it is student-centered. When adapting instruction, it is not only important to balance these two methods, but it is important to help students progress from didactic instruction to independent inquiry. While working from teacher-centered toward student-centered learning, the teacher needs to be aware of when or if students are ready for more independence. This requires that teachers know their students. Teachers must be tuned in to factors such as how their students learn, at what speed they learn, and what motivates them to learn. In health education PBL, the goal is for students to produce an outcome from their project while they learned about a health topic or skill along the way. Independent inquiry is likely to produce a student product.

Assessment Emphasis on Reflection and on Self and Peer Evaluation

Kokotsaki, Menzies, and Wiggins state that "evidence of progress needs to be regularly monitored and recorded" (2016, p. 274). In health PBL this can occur in several ways. We recommend that students keep a daily journal or other type of record that shows their progress. Peer evaluation summaries or progress notes could be recorded each day. The health teacher can have checkpoints during the process in which students must answer reflection questions about their progress, such as "Have you completed at least half of your project at this point?" "How many more resources do you need before you can move to the next step?" or "Have you started on the analysis portion?"

Student Choice and Autonomy

PBL allows students to choose how they will learn based on these things. However, the teacher must consider how to deliver the instruction so that all students have the opportunity to learn with their own style and abilities and even at their own pace. The first way we suggest is to allow students to choose their own projects. Some examples that students might choose are to develop a recycling project for their school, create a coronavirus PSA that can be shared with parents and the community, collect data from peers and develop a presentation, or work on a nutrition project that ends in healthy eating. As students choose their projects and begin working toward their outcome, they will develop goals for their projects, develop timelines for completion, determine who they might need to collaborate with along the way, and decide how they will investigate the problem they will be working on. All these components, giving students choice and autonomy, are key to PBL.

Entry Points

Developmental psychologist Howard Gardner (Edutopia 2009) discusses using multiple intelligences to enhance student learning. He believes that individual strengths in intelligences make a difference in the ability to learn and that teachers can use the strengths to connect to students and their style of learning. These become the entry point for a teacher to start the process of understanding a topic or skill. The key is to know your student and to know that each student will have a different entry point to develop an understanding of the topic you are teaching. For example, in Mr. Haun's class, he noticed that Claire is often drawing in class. She is likely to be a hands-on or tactile learner. It is important, then, that as Mr. Haun prepares the personal health unit and allows students to choose their projects, he should allow Claire to develop a project that is very hands-on. Gardner (1991) identifies five entry points to start learning any topic: aesthetic, narrative, logical or quantitative, foundational, and experimental or experiential. What follows are examples of what these might look like in health education.

Aesthetic

This entry point allows the student to use their senses. For example, during the stress management lesson, you would turn on relaxing music and have the students listen while they begin to plan their project for the unit. By using music, you engage those students who have a strong aesthetic entry point. They may actually choose to use music in their project to present their stress management technique to their peers.

Narrative

This entry point connects to students through a narrative or a story. For example, after playing music during the stress management lesson, you tell the students a story of a person who was very stressed and how they used art therapy to reduce the amount of stress they were under. This story might inspire them to write their own story about how stress management affects people.

Logical or Quantitative

This entry point uses data, numbers, or statistics so that students can connect to the topic. In the stress management lesson, you might present the number of people who suffer from stress in the United States. This allows students who are logical to consider surveying their peers and their level of stress for their project.

Foundational

This entry point connects with students through philosophical issues or big picture ideas that relate to the broader world. For example, you might briefly discuss how stress is linked to major health issues like cardiovascular disease and ask what some solutions might be to reduce this connection. The student project could look at worldwide stress and compare how different countries handle stress.

Experimental or Experiential

This entry point allows the student to experience the subject by doing. The teacher might actually have students lie on mats in the classroom and follow along with a progressive relaxation sequence from YouTube. Students with this learning style might choose a stress management technique and teach it to their peers.

Summary

As Mr. Haun recognized, students come to the classroom with a wide range of experiences, educational backgrounds, strengths, and ideas you can draw on in your health lessons. But it is essential to know the backgrounds of your students so you can meet them where they are on their curricular journey in health education. It is also important for you to know what they know, what their strengths are academically, and in what areas they need assistance. Armed with this knowledge, you and Mr. Haun can adapt your lessons to meet the strengths of each student.

Developing Students' Decision-Making Skills

It is the end of the school year, and as Mr. Dervent reflects on his health lessons, he realizes that his teaching features a major inconsistency. He always teaches decision-making to his students, yet he neither encourages nor requires that students use what they have been taught whenever they have to make decisions in class. This creates a credibility problem for him with his students. The bigger problem that he realizes is that this makes it much more unlikely that students will use these decision-making techniques when they are outside of school. He decides that in the coming year he is going to embed decision-making as a routine whenever students have to make decisions in his classes.

This chapter is not about creating a unit of instruction or scope and sequence of decision-making skills for K-12 students. For an example of that, see the Minnesota Department of Education resource on responsible decision-making (https://education.mn.gov). Instead, we focus on helping you identify knowledge, principles, and a specific model of decision-making that can be used across content and that students can use easily outside of school. We believe that all health education topics and skills lead to decision-making, and therefore it is important to embed it in each lesson and class period in some way.

Why Teach Decision-Making?

Our capacity to make decisions is critical to our success in life. We all make many decisions as we move through life. Over time we can learn, from trial and error, the value of some decisions versus others. Ideally, adolescents should not encounter many decisions, such as with sexual health and drug use, but the fact is that they frequently do. We expect adolescents to be able to cope with choices that life presents them on the basis of what they have learned at home or in school, yet most adolescents receive little or no formal training in the required decision-making skills other than in their health education curriculum each year.

Making decisions as an adolescent versus as an adult is more challenging because of at least two reasons. First, adolescents often have not had the benefit of experience that could inform their choices. Second, and most importantly, adolescents' brains are still developing. The American Academy of Child and Adolescent Psychiatry (2012) reports that the frontal cortex, the area of the brain that controls reasoning and helps you think before you act, changes and matures well into adulthood. The academy also reports that based on adolescents' stage of brain development, they are more likely to

- act on impulse,
- misread or misinterpret social cues and emotions,
- get into accidents of all kinds,
- get involved in fights, and
- engage in dangerous or risky behavior.

Adolescents are less likely to

- think before they act,
- pause to consider the potential consequences of their actions, and
- modify their dangerous or inappropriate behaviors.

None of this means, however, that adolescents cannot make good decisions. But it does mean they need guidance. As we will see in later in this chapter, guidance also involves allowing students to make mistakes so that they can learn from their mistakes.

What Do We Mean by Decision-Making?

Though often used interchangeably, *decision-making* and *problem-solving* are different tasks. A decision involves a number of skills that incorporate problem-solving, resulting in a choice from a variety of options. Problem-solving involves using available information to identify or design solutions to problems. Based on these definitions, problem-solving typically precedes decision-making. Most decision-making models incorporate the terms *decision-making* and *problem-solving* into their model for ease of understanding and presentation.

Decision-Making Model

Many decision-making models exist. What matters is that students use a model to inform their decisions. We use a model we have adapted from the work of Gregory (1991; Quist and Gregory, 2019). This model includes six steps in the practice of thoughtful decision-making.

1. *Framing*
   a. What must be decided and why?
   b. Can you frame the problem or decision as a choice?
   c. Be sure you do not simplify; include nuance in your discussion of the problem.
2. *Objectives*: What things do I or we care about that could be affected by this decision?
3. *Alternatives*: What alternatives can be considered?
4. *Consequences*: What are the likely consequences of different courses of action?
5. *Preferences*
   a. How do I or we feel about the trade-offs?
   b. What do I or we like best, all things considered?
6. *Adapting*: What could trigger me or us to reconsider, reassess, or adapt my or our behaviors?

This model is not designed to give the answers to students, but rather to help them consider alternatives and consequences, allowing them to make informed and thus defensible decisions. The model requires informed judgments that can stand the test of transparency, subject to peer and teacher review. But at the end of the day, answers to the questions in the model allow students to be independent and in control of their own decision-making. Using the model will not prevent students from making poor choices, ensure good outcomes, or change a student's core values. But it might prevent bad outcomes from occurring simply because the student is uninformed. One of the overarching goals of health education is to have better health outcomes throughout life; decision-making is the foundation for this goal.

Pedagogical Strategies and Considerations for Teaching Decision-Making

Some of the steps in the model require a different set of pedagogical strategies and considerations than are typically found in most classrooms. In this section we discuss important pedagogical strategies and considerations necessary when teaching decision-making.

Teach Students Active Listening Skills

Active listening is the skill of focusing on what a speaker is saying with the goal of understanding the message, comprehending the information, and responding thoughtfully. Active listeners use verbal and nonverbal techniques to show and keep their attention on the speaker. This not only supports the ability to focus on the speaker, but also helps the speaker see that you are focused and engaged. Active listening minimizes misunderstandings and creates respect. Active listening requires students to

- maintain eye contact with the speaker,
- not interrupt the speaker,
- repeat back key information to show they understand,
- ask questions to seek clarification, and
- listen to determine what the speaker is saying.

As students learn and practice decision-making in your classroom, it is important that the skill of active listening is part of the process. Listening actively to others can inform students and help them make good decisions, and the skill can be utilized in any or all of the six steps in the model. It is a skill that students must have for making health decisions throughout their lives.

Promote Mindfulness in Your Classroom

Though the term *mindfulness* has many definitions, Jon Kabat-Zinn, a pioneer of mindfulness practice, defines mindfulness as "paying attention in a particular way: on purpose, in the present moment, and non-judgmentally" (1994, p. 4). A growing number of schools are including lessons on mindfulness in their curricula because it counterbalances the anxiety and stress that so many students face and the poor self-control that they sometimes exhibit. Mindful thinking allows students to filter out distractions and reflect on the situation at hand. This is an important part of making decisions. Students must be able to determine what must be decided and why. If they are unable to focus on the entirety of the situation, they are less likely to make a good decision. Mindfulness techniques can reduce the negative effects of stress, increase students' abilities to stay engaged, help them stay on track academically, and help them avoid behavior problems, all of which require that they make decisions. Many resources for teaching mindfulness can be found online, in text, and in audio and video formats (e.g., www.waterford.org). Additionally, elementary and secondary lesson plans and mini curricula are available for different grade levels (e.g., Mindful Choices).

Let Students Live With Their Choices, and Avoid Rescuing Them

Decision-making grows stronger each time a student has to navigate the consequences of a good or a poor decision. Facing the natural consequences is how students gain experience. Consequences teach students the value of their decisions. In simple terms, this is experience, and learning from experience is an essential life skill. It is not just the skill of learning from experience that is important. Studies (Quist and Gregory 2019) show that student decision-making or choice is frequently listed as one of the most powerful motivating strategies a teacher can allow in the classroom. When given choices by teachers, students often perceive classroom activities as more important because they have some skin in the game as a result of their choices that commit them to particular actions.

Decision-Making Requires Practice

Decision-making is like playing sports. No one would expect a basketball player to become good after performing one layup. To have a good layup performance, the player must practice the layup hundreds, arguably thousands, of times. Decision-making also takes practice so that students repeatedly learn from their decisions. Decision-making can be made easier for students if they follow a common procedure or steps and if they have many opportunities to make defensible decisions. This is an essential reason decision-making should not be a unit of instruction, but rather a core skill that students use in all facets of the classroom and that is embedded in the content of health education daily.

Simulate Real-World Scenarios in the Classroom

Many decisions students need to make can be made easier if they have made these or similar decisions previously. Teaching strategies include approximating the scenario students might find themselves in and providing the opportunity to try out decisions and learn from the consequences and their peers. Such methods include the use of case studies, role-playing, debates, and projects (see PBL in chapter 12). Students learn best when they do, which means, in this case, when they make decisions about real situations. Covey (2006) suggests that adolescents regularly confront six classes of decisions:

1. Decisions about school, including their commitment to study and their future higher education expectations

2. Decisions about who their friends are and how to navigate friendships

3. Decisions about interacting positively with their parents

4. Decisions about dating and sex

5. Decisions about addictions, what they are, how they achieve power over people, and how to navigate social situations

6. Decisions about self-worth

We add a seventh:

7. Decisions about public health

All of these decisions occur in the content and context of health education. Constructing your teaching strategies around these themes when you cover different content creates recurring opportunities throughout your instruction to help students practice decision-making.

Recognize That Uncertainty Is Common to Decision-Making Scenarios

Uncertainty in life is like judging the weather forecast for the day. If the forecast predicts rain, a student will consider previous experiences and the current context with rain when deciding what to wear. For example, if a student is dropped off at school by the bus, the distance from the bus to the front door of the school and how hard it may rain will inform their judgment. On the other hand, if after school the student has to walk home and it may still be raining lightly, this might exert more influence over the decision. Students experience uncertainty when they believe that a number of potential decisions or solutions may be correct or when they choose actions based on often imperfect observations, with unknown outcomes. The goal is not to avoid, reduce, or fear uncertainty, but to better understand it and its implications for the decisions. Uncertainty is common, and because of this, what appears to be a simple decision might have more nuance. Examining the uncertainty and making decisions may not lead to good outcomes, but such examination does give the student the best way forward in that rationales drive the decision.

Revisit and Reflect

Students may not always be aware of what they are learning and experiencing. Teachers must create classroom cultures that cause students to be reflective. Reexamining choices and having students reflect on their actions are valuable activities. Fortunately, most decisions adolescents make are recurring ones, so teachers can always reexamine different decisions and have students reflect and discuss the consequences of their actions. Reflection in learning is necessary for students' improvement and in-depth learning, and is a process of personalizing and understanding the contents, process, and rationales for their decisions.

Teachers can do a lot to encourage reflection on decisions, including the following:

- Give students enough time to reflect
- Prompt students' reflection by asking questions that seek reasons and experience
- Provide some explanations to guide students' thought processes during explorations
- Provide a less structured learning environment that prompts students to explore what they think is important in their examination of their decisions
- Provide social-learning environments such as those inherent in peer-group work and small-group activities to allow students to see other points of view
- Encourage the use of reflective journaling so that students can write down their observations, provide reasons to support what they think, and show awareness of opposing positions and the weaknesses of their own positions

Summary

As Mr. Dervent reflects on his health lessons, he realizes that decision-making is a skill that needs practicing and that lies at the core of health education in order for students to make informed choices and to be independent consumers of health knowledge. This is the foundation of health literacy. In this chapter, we have argued that decision-making should not be a single unit of instruction, but rather the core skill that students learn and use regularly in their lives. We believe it should be the crux of health education content and lay the foundation for other skills identified in the National Health Education Standards. Health education at its best is not the provision of factual or research-based knowledge, but the interpretation and use of that knowledge by students best represented in their actions informed by their defensible decisions. Making health decisions requires informed, defensible judgments, but it also requires learning from experience and understanding that such learning may involve missteps along the way. Decision-making can be made easier for students if they follow a common procedure or steps.

Teaching decision-making will not prevent students from making poor choices, ensure good outcomes, or change a student's core values. But it may prevent bad outcomes from occurring as a result of being uninformed. As such, informed decision-making is one of the most important skills all of us can learn.

PART III

Growing as a Teacher

CHAPTER 14

Reflecting on Teaching

According to a famous saying, you can teach the same lesson a thousand times or you can teach a thousand different lessons. Mr. Santiago knows the reality of this saying well. He feels that he is teaching pretty much the way he has always taught. Yes, he is adding new ideas here and there, and he adjusts his lessons whenever the district modifies the curriculum, but he is frustrated that he is in this situation. Teaching is not exciting to him, and he feels like he is not progressing as a teacher.

The famous educator Madeline Hunter first made popular the idea that "teaching is decision making" (Hunter 1979). She argued that a teacher's decision-making includes applying professional and subject-specific knowledge and judgment in their work. Contemporary scholars (Verhoeven et al. 2019) emphasize that decisions by teachers are also influenced by sociocultural contexts, educational standards, and school values. Teaching, like other professions, has its own professional knowledge (e.g., psychology, sociology, pedagogy) and subject-specific knowledge (e.g., nutrition, mental health).

The professional and subject-specific knowledge require that teachers first know it and then use their judgment in applying it. The knowledge learned in university teacher education programs and in books like this one are grounded in the assumption that they work on paper. However, the professional judgments of teachers are not only informed by evidence-based practice, but they are also informed by craft knowledge. Craft knowledge is "that part of professional knowledge which teachers acquire primarily through their practical experience in the classroom" (Brown and McIntyre 1993, p. 17).

Our experience working with teachers over many decades and our research on this topic has taught us that effective teachers learn from experience. But learning from experience requires reflection and action.

Reflection

Though the word *reflection* has many definitions, forms, and foci, we define it in the context of teaching as the purposeful act of inquiry into your own behavior and students' behaviors, and the purpose is to improve your teaching and student learning. Reflection can take place before (e.g., reflecting on the previous lesson), during, or after the lesson. Reflection can also occur long after the event (e.g., reflecting on how you taught something last year). To reflect, you must first attend to the critical aspects of your teaching or student performance and then spend time reflecting on your observations.

Your reflection should be purposeful (i.e., you act on your findings), and it should result in maintenance of good teaching practices, refinement, and a focus on improving practices and those that are less effective. Think about a sculptor sculpting her clay (teaching behaviors and student learning) in different ways to produce the sculpture she envisions. In the context of teaching, you reflect on teaching behaviors and student learning different ways to produce the outcome you desire, student learning. Such reflection requires observation, judgment, and action. As teachers, you are expected to be intentional decision makers, and to that end, reflection is a critical teaching practice.

Reflection can be approached in many ways. Important considerations include the following:

1. Make notes in your lesson plan immediately following a lesson, when events are fresh in your mind. Chefs make many edits to recipes, changing the amount of ingredients or procedures in the margins. We think that lesson plans should be living documents as well, constantly modified with notes and comments in electronic documents or written on hard copies.

2. While you might make notes on your teaching, effective teachers also put aside time to reflect more deeply, particularly when your note at the end of lesson is something like, "Don't do it this way again." You will need time to research ways to do something differently the next time the lesson is taught.

3. After you write down your thoughts, make changes where necessary.

4. Reflection is not confined to a single lesson. Broader issues such as social justice or social and emotional learning (SEL) require more frequent reflection.

5. Not all reflection is focused on a lesson. Reflection can also be focused on other education issues like your mission statement, advocacy efforts, or social justice.

There is no one way to reflect, no one-size-fits-all strategy that works for all teachers. Different teachers use different methods or a combination of methods. Here are some common examples.

- *Talk with a peer or group of peers.* Reflection is helped by posing problems and asking questions. One good way to do this is with a peer or group of peers who meet regularly and can help unpack the issue you are reflecting on.

- *Ask students for their opinion.* It can be daunting to ask students how the lesson went, and you must be ready for the hard truth when asking for this information. You must never take it personally, but rather remember that this information is a way to reflect. Students can respond by writing on note cards or just in conversation. Getting students' opinions also engages them in the purpose of the lesson, and that is always a good thing.

- *Keep a reflection journal.* A reflection journal allows you to capture details of your teaching directly after class, which provides an ongoing narrative of your teaching across terms and years. Taking five or so minutes after class, write thoughts on the day's lesson (typing or handwriting works, although handwriting often supports better memory and reflection). You might reflect on the following questions: What went well today? What could I have done differently? How will I modify my instruction in the future?

- *Use teaching inventories.* Teaching inventories provide a sort of checklist to use as a self-check. They require you to respond to questions about your teaching practice and are usually designed to assess the extent to which particular teaching practices are used. They often consist of multiple-choice questions on a Likert scale and typically take less than 15 minutes to complete. You can find inventories online (www.developmentaldiscipline.com). Inventories are not something to be used regularly, but using them two or three times a year can be useful.

- *Video-record your teaching.* You can record your lessons using a camera, phone, or even wearable technologies such as GoPro. We favor cameras or phones because they focus clearly on you as the teacher. Observing your teaching can make visible to you things you would otherwise not see. Doing so can significantly increase your understanding of your teaching and the nuances of your lesson.

The Foci of Reflection

The topics that you reflect on might include the technical aspects of teaching (e.g., pedagogy), the influence of culture on your students (e.g., race, ethnicity, gender, class, religion, and ability) on learning, and issues of equity and social justice in your classroom and school. Pultorak (1996) discussed three foci for reflection:

1. *Technical rationality:* focuses on teacher competency and effectiveness
2. *Subjective reflection:* reveals personal bias and values based on personal perceptions
3. *Critical reflection:* considers the value of knowledge and moral or ethical dimensions of schooling

The sidebar provides examples of questions you might ask, but keep in mind that reflection is a habit and that it might focus on one or several questions in response to an event or as a general inquiry into your practice as a teacher.

Reflection Foci

Questions Focused on Technical Rationality

- What went well in the lesson?
- Did the students listen to the opinions, thoughts, and ideas of others?
- Were the students the center of the classroom discussion?
- Did students follow the classroom rules?
- Do the students interact well with each other?
- Did students follow the classroom rules?
- Did I have a positive demeanor during the lesson?
- Did the students work well with each other in their groups? Are there any changes I need to make with groups?
- Did the students accomplish my goals for the lesson? If not, what are my next steps?
- What method(s) of assessment did I use to determine the success, understanding, and progress of my students during this lesson?
- Did I provide opportunities for whole-group, small-group, and individual work?

- Did I modify my lesson based on the needs of the students?
- If I had to teach this lesson again, what would I do differently?

Questions Focused on Subjective Reflection

- What were my goals for this lesson? That is, what did I want the students to know, understand, and be able to do as a result of this lesson?
- Why did I plan this learning experience as a way to achieve my goals?
- Was I prepared for today's lesson? Did I have all my materials prepared and organized?
- How do I think I handled any classroom disruptions or student behavior issues?
- To what extent were my students engaged in the lesson?
- Did the students appear interested in and excited about the lesson?
- What did I do to engage the students or get them excited at the beginning of the lesson?
- Did the students accomplish my goals for the lesson? If not, what are my next steps?
- What was the most challenging part of this lesson?
- Did the students do most of the talking, or did I?
- Do I feel there were any missed opportunities in this lesson when I could have gone into more depth or expanded the lesson in some way?
- Did any students struggle with this lesson? What are some strategies or activities I can use that might help them master the content and skills in the lesson?
- Were accommodations provided for both high achievers and struggling students?

Questions Focused on Critical Reflection

- Who benefits in this situation?
- Whose voices are being omitted?
- For what purpose is the content being taught?
- Who is advantaged, disadvantaged, or excluded by the teaching of this content?
- What are the messages being conveyed by the teaching of this content in this way?
- What is not being taught on this topic?

Summary

If Mr. Santiago wants to grow as a teacher, he needs to do more than incidentally reflect on his teaching. He needs to engage in regular and systematic evaluation of his teaching. He can explore different methods and select questions that are most relevant for himself and his classes. Then he can act on his reflections, which include continuing to use his questioning techniques or changing how he presents his lessons to address the cultural diversity of his students. What matters here is that he develops a habit of reflection. With practice he will not only get better at attending to the critical aspects of his teaching because he is more reflective and intentional, but he will get better at determining which questions to ask and which actions to follow up on.

Being a Professional

There were once two teachers. Both had graduated from good health education programs, and they were both fortunate enough to obtain jobs in similar public middle schools. As their careers advanced, noticeable changes occurred in each teacher. Mr. Hernandez's career was characterized by teaching his classes, attending school meetings and required professional development activities, and engaging in extracurricular activities such as coaching. However, if you attended Mr. Hernandez's classes throughout his career, for the most part, his pedagogy remained unchanged, and his lessons were more similar than different. In fact, he was at his best as a teacher in the first five years of his teaching. He remained mostly unaffected by the changes of the field of health education. Ms. Jobert, on the other hand, continued to grow throughout her career. She helped the district design the health curriculum, and she was active in the state professional association. She attended conferences whether they were supported by her school or not, and she actively read and searched the internet for ways to improve her teaching of health. She also met monthly with some peers to discuss teaching in general and teaching health in particular.

In our experience many teachers fit into one of these two modes of professional growth. Clearly, we encourage Ms. Jobert's mode. But when we have asked teachers like Mr. Hernandez why they didn't engage in professional development activities to the extent that Ms. Jobert did, a common answer is that they expected the district to provide such opportunities. We agree that districts should provide frequent and meaningful professional development opportunities, but even with such opportunities, it is incumbent on each of us to step up and engage in developing our expertise.

What It Means to Be a Professional

Teachers have professional, specialized knowledge as is the case with lawyers, physicians, engineers, and psychologists. This knowledge is first acquired in the teacher education program, but it is developed further and refined throughout one's career as a result of experience and through formal and informal professional development. You are always a student learning about teaching and whom you are teaching. A key consideration of being a professional also includes the application of professional knowledge, self-evaluation, adherence to codes of conduct, advocacy for their field, and engagement in continuous professional development.

Application of Professional Knowledge

Classrooms often display the following characteristics:

- *Multidimensionality:* many events and tasks occur in a typical lesson (e.g., student questioning, student misbehavior, student misunderstanding)
- *Simultaneity:* many of these events occur at the same time
- *Immediacy:* many tasks require an immediate response (e.g., student misunderstanding or misbehavior)
- *Unpredictability:* some events occur unexpectedly (e.g., interruptions such as requests to leave the room for appointments elsewhere in the school)
- *Publicness:* these events are seen by everyone in the class
- *History:* students have a history with the subject and the teacher (Doyle 1986)

Because of these characteristics, a one-size-fits-all or prescriptive approach to teaching cannot be used. Teachers must apply and adapt their professional knowledge and prowess to meet the needs of the students in their classes and in doing so, must make decisions frequently and often very quickly. Applying professional knowledge regularly to guide decision-making increases the likelihood of student learning.

Another consideration is that health education content knowledge is evolving continually and, as such, it requires that teachers are up to date with their knowledge. Likely, no other subject in school so frequently requires teachers to respond to student questions, "I don't know the answer, but I will follow up on it and get back to you tomorrow" or "I don't know the answer, so I want everyone—myself included—to research it tonight and report back tomorrow on what you find out." It is simply not possible to know everything that is going on in the world of health education. But it is also true that teachers have a professional responsibility to engage in professional development and research to stay up to date with current trends in the field. For example, in chapter 1 we discussed the 10 big ideas of health education. Many of these ideas are unknown to teachers if they have not been active in their professional learning.

What You Can Do

In order to grow your professional knowledge, we recommend a few things. Some ideas are discussed elsewhere throughout this book, such as reflecting with peers (see chapter 14), but the following list provides additional ideas that will enhance your professional knowledge.

- Subscribe to professional journals, and delve into the latest research and teaching tips. In health education, we recommend the *Journal of School Health*, the *American Journal of Health Education*, and *Health Education Journal*.

- Create a professional learning plan (PLP). This can be a chart with events and dates mapped out, or it could be a journal or calendar that you keep with reminders of things to do that enhance your knowledge.

- Obtain continuing education units (CEUs) regularly. These are sometimes offered by your district or state, but other times you must seek them out. They can be obtained from the journal articles you read, at conferences you attend, or from online webinars in which you participate.

- Take additional college classes in your areas of weakness. After self-evaluating and determining the areas in which you need to take action, see if your local university offers classes in that area, and sign up.

Teacher Evaluation of Their Practice

In chapter 14 we discussed how to reflect on three broad, important foci of reflection: technical rationality, subjective reflection, and critical reflection. Reflective teachers are thoughtful and critical about their teaching. Reflection is a growth strategy that is an important part of being a teacher, and we encourage you to set up ways to do this with yourself and peers.

What You Can Do

- Engage in regular evaluation of your formative and summative assessments (see chapter 7). Analyze your objectives, then your assessment, and finally your instruction and content.

- Examining your objectives, assessment, instruction, and content allows you to determine if your objectives are aligned with standards and big ideas, if your assessment measured what you described as your objectives, and if the instruction and content you used were aligned with your assessment tasks.

Lortie (1975) observed that teaching is often viewed as more of an individualistic rather than a collaborative activity. Health education teachers often work in isolated settings because they may be the only health educator in a school. A solution is to connect with health educators in other buildings and other teachers of different subject matters. Participate in formal and informal professional development communities, also referred to as professional learning communities or communities of practice. Within these communities, a group of teachers meets regularly throughout the year, whether in person or virtually, to discuss issues of teaching, building on the ideas and practices discussed in the group. They require engagement and collaboration on common challenges in teaching and are most often designed to improve student learning. These groups exemplify teachers accepting responsibility for their own professional growth and knowledge.

Adherence to Codes of Conduct

All professionals have codes of conduct. Professional organizations such as teachers' unions and most states have codes of conduct for teachers. Read through these codes periodically for clarity on the scope of the teacher's role. In their study of ethical concerns of teachers, Barrett et al. (2006) identified three broad domains of concerns of teachers. The first is student–teacher boundary violations (i.e., nonprofessional relationships with students). Such relationships represent a conflict of interest for teachers and pose a significant risk for emotional or physical harm.

The second domain of concern is carelessness in interpersonal behavior and in instruction, such as gossiping to colleagues about students and speaking disparagingly about other teachers to colleagues, coming to class unprepared, and engaging in activities in the classroom that are not relevant to instruction. Each of these have professional, employment, and legal consequences.

The third domain of concern is subjectivity in grading and instruction. Teachers are under considerable pressure relative to grading, as Barrett et al. (2006, p. 431) note:

> For example, more than 25% of teachers reported that teachers often raise grades due to parental pressure, and more than 80% of teachers viewed this as a serious violation of professional

standards. Similarly, more than 25% of teachers reported that teachers often give children higher grades if they personally like the students, and almost 85% viewed this behavior as a serious violation of teacher ethics.

In the study by Barrett et al. (2006), teachers rated boundary violations as the most serious but the least common, and carelessness in behavior as the most common but least serious violation. Regardless of the perception of violations, teachers must abide by a code of conduct that reduces the risk of issues with students, learning, and colleagues that would have a negative impact on their career.

What You Can Do

- Become a member of your professional association. In health education, we recommend several, including SHAPE America, National Association of Health and Kinesiology, and your state health and physical education associations (e.g., CASHAPE).

- Be transparent in your teaching with students, parents, and administrators so that nothing is hidden from stakeholders. For example, you might allow a time for parents to view your curriculum prior to teaching. You might have a class website that discusses your policies for classroom management. It might also mean that you turn in a block plan to your administrator so that they are aware of your teaching intentions.

- Be familiar with the codes of conduct. See the National Education Association code of conduct (www.nea.org) and your state's teaching code of conduct (e.g., Ohio's at https://education.ohio.gov).

- Know your district's procedures for self-reporting or reporting observed violations of ethical misconduct.

Advocacy for Health Education

Teachers are expected to be agents of change for their subject matter and students: "Teaching at its core is a moral profession. Scratch a good teacher and you will find a moral purpose" (Fullan 1993, p. 12). The best advocacy a teacher can engage in is to be a caring and effective teacher. This includes sharing the importance of your subject matter with students, their parents, other teachers in your school, and administrators. All health educators should have two goals for local advocacy efforts. First, increase the students', parents', other teachers', and administrators' awareness of the importance of health education. Second, report on the accomplishments of your students.

What You Can Do

- Use credible data to show that your teaching is accomplishing your goals. One approach is to present test scores, project or assignment scores, and the average and range of student grades. Other approaches include demonstrating that your students know and can make a difference with their knowledge by applying it in real-world contexts. This can include engaging in project-based learning in the school (e.g., courtesy and respect; handwashing and coughing etiquette; student- or teacher-led yoga, meditation, or mindfulness for stress reduction) or community (e.g., helping community agencies enhance their websites or working on community goals on oral health, smoking, and healthy eating).

- Use schoolwide announcements to promote health-related activities (e.g., lunchtime walking program, stress reduction sessions).

- Host parent nights at the beginning of the year to describe your curriculum and outcomes and to show student work from previous years.

- Use parent–teacher conferences to display student work on bulletin boards, PowerPoints, and other media sources.

- Keep a class or subject website where you post student videos or projects.

- Regularly send home health newsletters that include discussion points for families. Increase the probability they will be read by having students contribute to the design.

- Include in homework age-appropriate conversation prompts with parents and siblings.

- Create partnerships with health-related groups (e.g., medical communities) or businesses (e.g., local workout facilities) to sponsor projects. Make formal presentations to these groups.

- Use social media, radio, and television to promote district agendas for health education.

- Present to your local school board highlights of what you do in your health education program. Use the above ideas as evidence, and do not be afraid to include a list of materials and resources you need.

Engagement in district, regional, state, and national efforts and associations is one way to familiarize yourself with the how-to of advocacy, and then you can get involved in ongoing advocacy efforts. As a beginning teacher you might start more locally, whereas more experienced teachers might choose to engage in state- or national-level activities. There is strength in numbers, and adding yourself to the numbers of those who are doing this work is important.

Engagement in Continuous Professional Development

We use the term *continuous professional development* rather than the more common *continuing professional development* to emphasize that professional development does not mean simply continuing past one's teacher education training, but rather that it is a frequently recurring effort grounded in inquiry into the practice of teaching. The terms *frequently* and *recurring* imply that professional development is an active process: it is proactive and ongoing, and it will produce outcomes, but it is not a destination.

What You Can Do

- Attend local, state, and national professional conferences (e.g., SHAPE America annual convention).

- Inquire into existing professional development communities in your school or district, or national or global online communities. Alternatively, start one yourself.

- Find mentors in and out of your subject matter whom you can bounce ideas off of and turn to for advice.

- Find several go-to sources for health education that you can routinely visit for updates on teaching health and to improve your professional knowledge. These sources might include the following:
  - SHAPE America (www.shapeamerica.org)
  - Centers for Disease Control and Prevention (www.cdc.gov)
  - Publishers such as Human Kinetics
  - Health education blogs such as *#slowchathealth* (https://slowchat health.com) and *Health Teacher* (https://thehealthteacher.com)
  - Health teacher websites such as Support Real Teachers (www.supportrealteachers.org) and Life Is the Future (https://lifeis thefuture.com/)

Summary

The responsibility for being a professional is on you. It is not something you call yourself, but rather it is defined by your actions and how others view your actions relative to your professional conduct. Central to the notion of being a professional is the application of your professional knowledge to improve instruction and student learning, self-evaluation of your practice with the goal of improving your lessons and curriculum, adhering to codes of conduct, advocating for your field, and engaging in continuous professional development throughout your career. In short, we want the field to consist of motivated people like Ms. Jobert, not complacent people like Mr. Hernandez.

Final Thoughts

We began this book with the statement that teachers make a difference. We conclude with this observation: Teachers make a difference if they use the skills of their profession. In this book we used the concept of core practices, that is, knowledge and skills that are central to effective teaching. These core practices are often referred to as best practices in teaching. Research supports their use, and importantly, they affect student learning. However, their use creates organization and direction for teaching, and over time, they allow teachers to do what they most love: teaching students and seeing them learn without being distracted by organization and management issues that interfere with doing their job. As a result of how the core practices are used by teachers, they also lead students to take on more responsibility for their own learning, resulting in student empowerment.

We wrote this book because we believe that health education in K-12 schools is suffering, not because teachers are not well intentioned or lacking in subject matter knowledge, but because overwhelming evidence points to a lack of core practices being taught and used by teachers in the health classroom. It is our hope that this book contributes to the development and support of teachers as they teach our children and youth.

References

PREFACE

Ball, D.L., Sleep, L., Boerst, T., & Bass, H. (2009). Combining the development of practice and the practice of development in teacher education. *Elementary School Journal, 109*(5), 458-474.

Fogo, B. (2014). Core practices for teaching history: The results of a Delphi panel survey. *Theory & Research in Social Education, 42*, 151-196. doi:10.1080/00933104.2014.902781.

Grossman, P., Hammerness, K., & McDonald, M. (2009). Redefining teaching, reimagining teacher education. *Teachers and Teaching, 15*, 273-289. doi:10.1080/13540600902875340

Kloser, M. (2014). Identifying a core set of science teaching practices: A Delphi expert panel approach. *Journal of Research in Science Teaching, 51*, 1185-1217. doi:10.1002/tea.21171

Schneider Kavanagh, S.; Shahan, E., & Morrison, D. (2017). Core practices of teaching: A primer. http://tfajaxelementary.weebly.com/uploads/6/5/7/8/ 6578913/core_practice_primer.pdf.

Windschitl, M., Thompson, J., & Braaten, M. (2018). *Ambitious science teaching*. Boston, MA: Harvard Education.

CHAPTER 1

Ball, D.L., Sleep, L., Boerst, T., & Bass, H. (2009). Combining the development of practice and the practice of development in teacher education. *Elementary School Journal, 109*(5), 458-474.

CDC (2015). Whole School, Whole Community, Whole Child (WSCC). www.cdc.gov/healthyschools/wscc/index.htm

CDC (2018). Characteristics of an Effective Health Education Curriculum. www.cdc.gov/healthyschools/sher/characteristics/index.htm

Fogo, B. (2014). Core practices for teaching history: The results of a Delphi panel survey. *Theory & Research in Social Education, 42*, 151-196. doi:10.1080/00933104.2014.902781

Forzani, F. (2014). Understanding "core practices" and "practice-based" teacher education: Learning from the past. *Journal of Teacher Education, 65*, 357-368. doi:10.1177/0022487114533800.

Grossman, P., Hammerness, K., & McDonald, M. (2009). Redefining teaching, reimagining teacher education. *Teachers and Teaching, 15*, 273-289. doi:10.1080/13540600902875340

Hattie, J. 2009. *Visible Learning: A Synthesis of Over 800 Meta-Analyses Relating to Achievement*. London: Routledge.

Kloser, M. (2014). Identifying a core set of science teaching practices: A Delphi expert panel approach. *Journal of Research in Science Teaching, 51*, 1185-1217. doi:10.1002/tea.21171

Marzano, R.J. (2010). *On excellence in teaching*. Bloomington, IN: Solution Tree Press.

Marzano, R.J., J.S. Marzano, and D.J. Pickering. 2003. *Classroom Management That Works: Research-Based Strategies for Every Teacher*. Alexandria, VA: Association for Supervision and Curriculum Development.

McDonald, M., Kazemi, E., & Kavanagh, S. S. (2013). Core practices and pedagogies of teacher education: A call for a common language and collective activity. *Journal of Teacher Education, 64*, 378-386.

Millican, J.S., & Helweh-Forrester, S.H. (2018). Core practices in music teaching: A Delphi expert panel survey." Journal of Music Teacher Education, 27(3), 155-168. doi:10.1177/1057083717736243

Schneider Kavanagh, S.; Shahan, E., & Morrison, D. (2017). Core practices of teaching: A primer, http://tfajaxelementary.weebly.com/uploads/6/5/7/8/ 6578913/core_prac tice_primer.pdf .

Windschitl, M., Thompson, J., & Braaten, M. (2018). *Ambitious science teaching.* Boston, MA: Harvard Education.

CHAPTER 2

BC's Curriculum. n.d. "Physical Health and Education." Accessed March 26, 2021. https://curriculum.gov.bc.ca/curriculum/physical-health-education.

Mitchell, I., Keast, S., Panizzon, D., & Mitchell, J. (2016). Using "big ideas" to enhance teaching and student learning. *Teachers and Teaching*, 1-15. doi:10.1080/13540602. 2016.1218328

Wiggins, G. (2010). What's my job? Defining the role of the classroom teacher. In R. J. Marzano (Ed.), *On Excellence in Teaching* (10th ed., pp. 7-29). Bloomington, IN: Solution Tree Press.

Windschitl, M., Thompson, J., & Braaten, M. (2018). *Ambitious Science Teaching.* Boston, MA: Harvard Education.

CHAPTER 3

Maryland comprehensive health education framework. http://marylandpublicschools. org/about/Documents/DCAA/Health/HealthEducationFramework_Final.pdf

Wiggins, G., and J. McTighe. (1998). *Understanding by Design.* Alexandria, VA: Association for Supervision and Curriculum Development.

CHAPTER 4

Wiggins, G., and J. McTighe. (1998). *Understanding by Design.* Alexandria, VA: Association for Supervision and Curriculum Development.

CHAPTER 5

Bruner, J. (1960). *The Process of Education.* Cambridge, MA: Harvard University Press.

Ma, L. 1999. *Knowing and Teaching Elementary Mathematics.* Mahwah, NJ: Lawrence Erlbaum Associates.

Madison Public Schools. n.d. "Health." Accessed March 30, 2021. www.madison.k12. ct.us/uploaded/docs/CurriculumGuides/Health_curr.pdf

National Research Council. 2007. *Taking Science to School: Learning and Teaching Science in Grades K-8.* Washington, DC: The National Academies Press. https://doi. org/10.17226/11625.

Popham, W.J. 2007. "All About Accountability: The Lowdown on Learning Progressions." *Educational Leadership* 64 (7): 83-84.

CHAPTER 6

Ball, D.L. 1990. "Prospective Elementary and Secondary Teachers' Understanding of Division." *Journal for Research in Mathematics Education* 21 (2): 132-144.

Clark, R.E., P.A. Kirschner, and J. Sweller. 2012. "Putting Students on the Path to Learning: The Case for Fully Guided Instruction." *American Educator* 36 (Spring): 6-11.

Illinois State University. n.d. "Revised Bloom's Taxonomy." Accessed March 31, 2021. https://education.illinoisstate.edu/downloads/casei/5-02-Revised%20Blooms.pdf.

Rosenshine, B. 2012. "Principles of Instruction: Research-Based Strategies That All Teachers Should Know." *American Educator* 36 (Spring): 12-19, 39.

University of Iowa Center for Teaching. n.d. "Using Concept Maps as Teaching Tools." Accessed March 31, 2021. https://teach.its.uiowa.edu/sites/teach.its.uiowa.edu/files/docs/docs/Concept_Maps_as_Teaching_Tools_ed.pdf.

CHAPTER 7

The Council of Chief State School Officers. 2018. *Revising the Definition of Formative Assessment.* https://ccsso.org/sites/default/files/2018-06/Revising%20the%20Definition%20of%20Formative%20Assessment.pdf.

Ellens, J. 2019. "8 Quiz Ideas Your Audience Will Love + 61 Proven Quiz Titles." Lead Quizzes. www.leadquizzes.com/blog/quiz-ideas-and-titles.

The Teacher Toolkit. n.d. "Entry Ticket." Accessed March 31, 2021. www.theteachertoolkit.com/index.php/tool/entry-ticket

The Teacher Toolkit. n.d. "Exit Ticket." Accessed March 31, 2021. www.theteachertoolkit.com/index.php/tool/exit-ticket.

TeachThought. 2020. "27 Simple Ways to Check for Understanding." www.teachthought.com/pedagogy/27-simple-ways-check-understanding.

University of Iowa Center for Teaching. n.d. "Using Concept Maps as Teaching Tools." Accessed March 31, 2021. https://teach.its.uiowa.edu/sites/teach.its.uiowa.edu/files/docs/docs/Concept_Maps_as_Teaching_Tools_ed.pdf.

CHAPTER 8

Alter, P., & Haydon, T. (2017). Characteristics of effective classroom rules: A review of the literature. *Teacher Education and Special Education, 40*(2), 114-127.

Doyle, W. (1986). Classroom organization and management. In M.C. Wittrock (Ed.), *Handbook of Research on Teaching* (pp. 392–431). New York, NY: Macmillan.

Ingersoll, R., & Smith, T. (2004). "Do teacher induction and mentoring matter?" *NASSP Bulletin, 88* (638), 28-40.

Siedentop, D., Hastie, P.A., & van der Mars, H. (2020). *Complete Guide to Sport Education.* Champaign, IL: Human Kinetics.

CHAPTER 9

The Inspired Educator. 2018. "8 Quick Relationship Building Activities." http://the-inspired-educator.com/8-quick-relationship-building-activities.

Klocke, A., and S. Stadtmüller. 2019. "Social Capital in the Health Development of Children." *Child Indicators Research,* 12, 1167-1185. https://doi.org/10.1007/s12187-018-9583-y.

National Center for Children in Poverty. n.d. "Young Child Risk Calculator." Accessed April 1, 2021. www.nccp.org/tools/risk/.

Sander, T.H., and R.D. Putnam. 1999. "Rebuilding the Stock of Social Capital." *School Administrator* 56 (8): 28-33.

CHAPTER 10

Facing History and Ourselves. n.d. "Socratic Seminar." Accessed April 2, 2021. www.facinghistory.org/resource-library/teaching-strategies/socratic-seminar.

Gonzalez, J. 2015. "The Big List of Class Discussion Strategies." www.cultofpedagogy.com/speaking-listening-techniques/.

Grossman, P. (Ed.). (2018). *Teaching Core Practices in Teacher Education*. Cambridge, MA: Harvard Education Press.

Witherspoon, M., Sykes, G., & Bell, C. (2016). *Leading a Classroom Discussion: Definition, supportive evidence, and measurement of the* ETS® *National Observational Teaching Examination (NOTE) assessment series* (Research Memorandum No. RM-16-09). Princeton, NJ: Educational Testing Service.

CHAPTER 11

Hattie, J., and H. Timperley. 2007. "The Power of Feedback." *Review of Educational Research* 77, 81-112.

CHAPTER 12

Buck Institute for Education. n.d. "Gold Standard PBL: Project Based Teaching Practices." Accessed April 5, 2021. www.pblworks.org/what-is-pbl/gold-standard-teaching-practices.

Edutopia. 2009. "Big Thinkers: Howard Gardner on Multiple Intelligences." Brain-Based Learning. www.edutopia.org/multiple-intelligences-howard-gardner-video.

Gardner, H. 1991. *The Unschooled Mind*. New York: Basic Books.

High Quality Project Based Learning. n.d. "HQPBL." Accessed April 5, 2021. https://hqpbl.org/.

Kokotsaki, D., V. Menzies and A. Wiggins. 2016. "Project-Based Learning: A Review of the Literature." *Improving Schools* 19 (3), 267-277. https://doi.org/10.1177/1365480216659733.

Tomlinson, C.A., and T. Moon. 2013. "Differentiation and Classroom Assessment." In *SAGE Handbook of Research on Classroom Assessment*, edited by J.H. McMillian, 415-430. Los Angeles: SAGE.

CHAPTER 13

American Academy of Child and Adolescent Psychiatry. 2011. "The Teen Brain: Behavior, Problem Solving, and Decision Making." Facts for Families. www.aacap.org/AACAP/Families_and_Youth/Facts_for_Families/FFF-Guide/The-Teen-Brain-Behavior-Problem-Solving-and-Decision-Making-95.aspx

Covey, S. 2006. *The 6 Most Important Decisions You'll Ever Make*. New York: Simon and Schuster.

Gregory, R. 1991. Critical Thinking for Environmental Health Risk Education. *Health Education Quarterly* 18 (3): 273-284.

Kabat-Zinn, J. 1994. *Wherever You Go, There You Are: Mindfulness Meditation in Everyday Life*. New York: Hyperion.

Minnesota Department of Education. n.d. "Responsible Decision-Making." Accessed April 5, 2021. https://education.mn.gov/mdeprod/groups/communications/documents/hiddencontent/bwrl/mdcz/~edisp/mde073493.pdf.

Quist, A., and R. Gregory. 2019. "Teaching Decision-Making Skills in the Classroom." The Arithmetic of Compassion. www.arithmeticofcompassion.org/blog/2019/5/1/teaching-decision-making-skills-in-the-classroom?rq=decision.

CHAPTER 14

Brown, S., and D. McIntyre. 1993. *Making Sense of Teaching*. Buckingham, UK: Open University Press.

Developmental Discipline. 2006. "Teacher Self-Reflection Inventory." http://developmentaldiscipline.com/Developmental_Discipline/Conference_Handouts_files/%20Self-Reflection%20Inventory.pdf.

Hunter, M. 1979. Teaching Is Decision Making. *Educational Leadership* 37 (1): 62-67.

Pultorak, E.G. 1996. "Following the Developmental Process of Reflection in Novice Teachers: Three Years of Investigation." *Journal of Teacher Education* 47, 283-291.

Verhoeven, M., Poorthuis, A.M.G., & Volman, M. 2019. The Role of School in Adolescents' Identity Development. A Literature Review." *Educational Psychologyl Review* 31, 35-63. https://doi.org/10.1007/s10648-018-9457-3

CHAPTER 15

Barrett, D.E., K.N. Headley, B. Stovall, and J.C. Witte. 2006. "Teachers' Perceptions of the Frequency and Seriousness of Violations of Ethical Standards." *The Journal of Psychology* 140 (5): 421-433.

Centers for Disease Control and Prevention. 2021. "Whole School, Whole Community, Whole Child (WSCC)." CDC Healthy Schools. www.cdc.gov/healthyschools/wscc/index.htm.

Doyle, W. 1986. "Classroom Organization and Management." In *Handbook of Research on Teaching*, edited by M.C. Wittrock, 392-431. New York: Macmillan.

Fullan, M.G. 1993. "Why Teachers Must Become Change Agents." *Educational Leadership* 50 (6): 12-17.

The Health Teacher. n.d. "Home." Accessed April 7, 2021. https://thehealthteacher.com/.

Lortie, D. 1975. *Schoolteacher: A Sociological Study*. London: University of Chicago Press.

National Education Association. 2020. "Code of Ethics for Educators." www.nea.org/resource-library/code-ethics-educators.

Ohio State Board of Education. 2019. "Licensure Code of Professional Conduct for Ohio Educators." Ohio Department of Education. http://education.ohio.gov/getattachment/Topics/Teaching/Educator-Conduct/Licensure-Code-of-Professional-Conduct-for-Ohio-Ed/Licensure-Code-of-Professional-Conduct.pdf.aspx?lang=en-US.

SHAPE America. n.d. "School Health Education: Guidance Documents & Position Statements." Accessed April 7, 2021. www.shapeamerica.org/advocacy/positionstatements/health/default.aspx?hkey=37a633ba-1f2a-4bd8-bf12-94c47b476693.

#slowchathealth. n.d. "Home." Accessed April 7, 2021. https://slowchathealth.com/.

Support Real Teachers. n.d. "Online Resources for Health, Fitness, and Nutrition." Accessed April 7, 2021. www.supportrealteachers.org/resources-for-health-fitness-and-nutrition.html.

Index

About the Authors

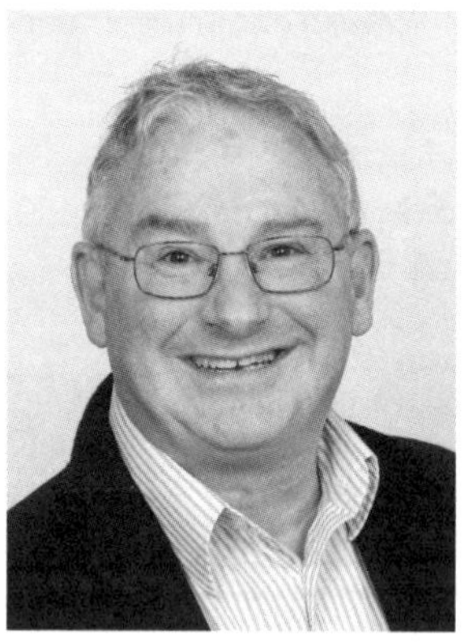

Dr. Phillip Ward, a leading scholar in the area of core practices for health education, is a professor of kinesiology in the department of human sciences at The Ohio State University. He teaches courses in health and physical education teacher education. He has authored multiple books in health and physical education, including another Human Kinetics text, *Effective Physical Education Content and Instruction* (2018). He is also coauthor of key policy documents for SHAPE America (Society of Health and Physical Educators) and the National Association for Kinesiology in Higher Education (NAKHE), and he has authored or coauthored more than 130 research papers and book chapters and has presented over 150 papers at international, national, and state conferences. Dr. Ward regularly reviews the standards for health education teacher education programs for the state of Ohio.

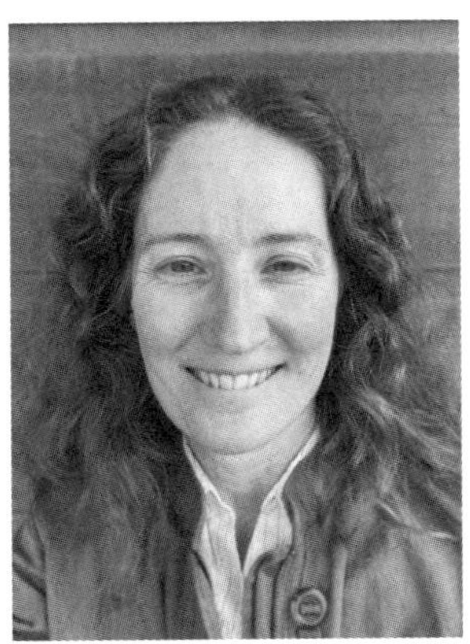

Dr. Shonna Snyder is an associate professor and past program coordinator of health and physical education at Gardner-Webb University in North Carolina. She has been teaching health education methodology courses in higher education since 2005. She is a coauthor of "Appropriate Practices in School-Based Health Education," a key guidance document in health education from SHAPE America (Society of Health and Physical Educators), and of "Student Recruitment for Physical Education and Health Education Teacher Education Programs," a key policy document for SHAPE America and the National Association for Kinesiology in Higher Education. She has also recently coauthored "Health Education/SEL Crosswalk: Aligning the National Health Education Standards With CASEL Social and Emotional Learning Competencies" (SHAPE America). Dr. Snyder has 12 peer-reviewed publications, has presented at the national and state levels, and regularly reviews textbooks for several health textbook publishers as well as journal articles for journal publications. She has authored blogs and webinars and been a guest speaker in many educational settings. She recently served on the North Carolina SHAPE (NCAAHPERD-SM) board of directors and is helping develop the North Carolina SHAPE journal. She is also serving as the SHAPE America Health Education Council chair and has been a member of the Health Education Council, Health Literacy Task Force, SHAPE America–NAKHE HETE/PETE Program Recruitment Task Force, School Health Education Task Force, and the Annual Program Planning Committee.

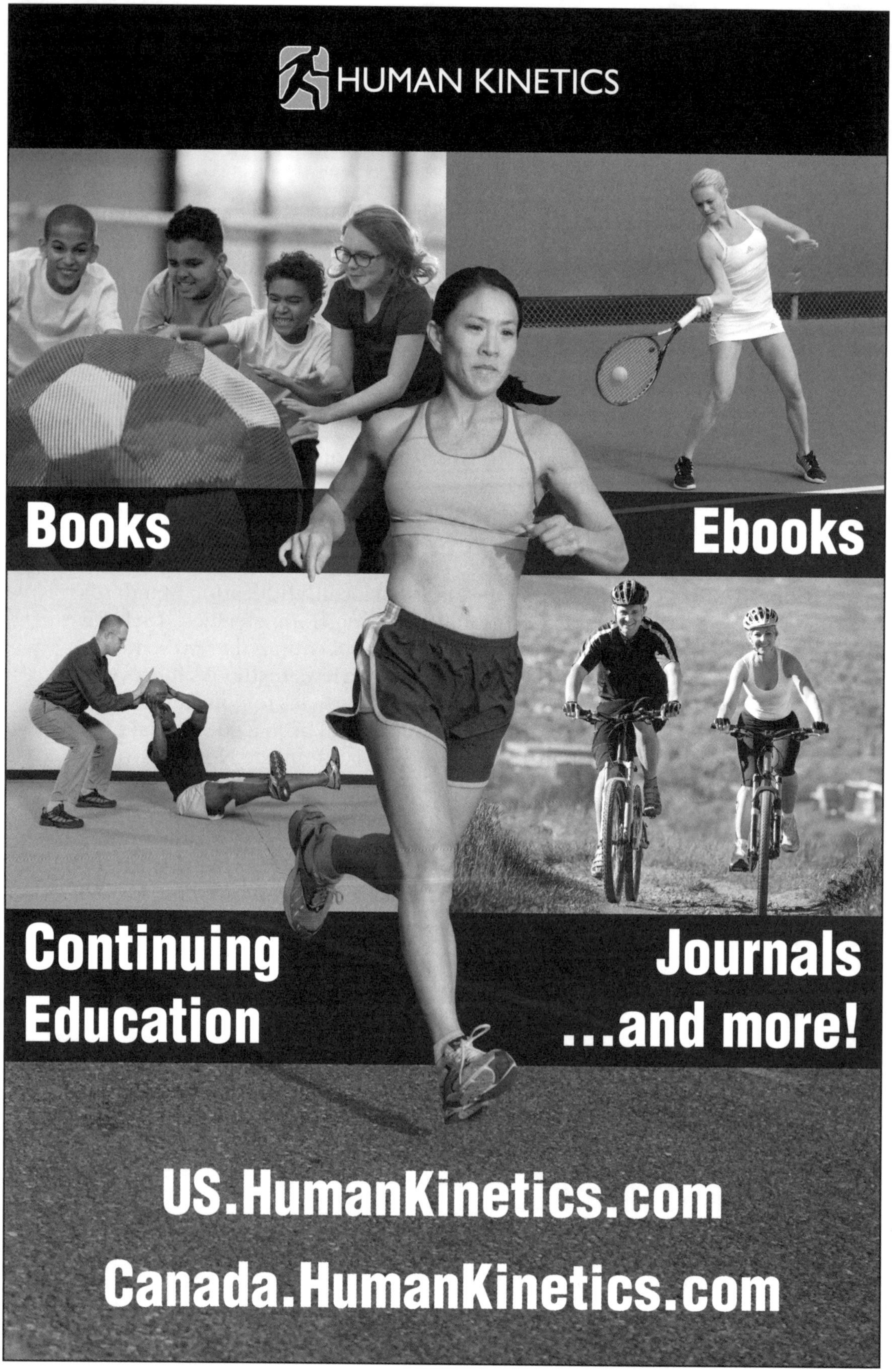

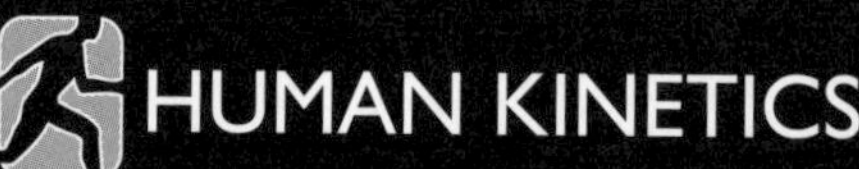

HUMAN KINETICS
Books
Ebooks
Continuing Education
Journals ...and more!
US.HumanKinetics.com
Canada.HumanKinetics.com